THE
Fast and fresh
ANTI-INFLAMMATORY
COOKBOOK

with **150** DELICIOUS RECIPES TO
REDUCE INFLAMMATION,
RESTORE YOUR HEALTH &
MAKE YOU FEEL AMAZING

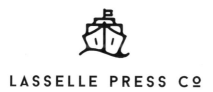

LASSELLE PRESS Cₒ

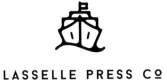

LASSELLE PRESS C<u>o</u>

ISBN-13: 978-1911364023
ISBN-10: 1911364022

CONTENTS

INTRODUCTION

Welcome to The Fast and Fresh Anti-Inflammatory Cookbook! Chances are you've picked this up because you, or someone you know, may be experiencing the uncomfortable and painful symptoms that come with inflammation.

You are not alone in experiencing these symptoms of inflammation, or perhaps knowing somebody who does. Inflammation is part of our body's healthy response system but what happens when we experience extreme pain and further problems? That's when the normal inflammation process has gone wrong. This book gives you an overview of the key aspects of chronic inflammation, in order to give you a better understanding of the causes, symptoms and the various diseases and illnesses which have been linked to chronic inflammation, such as diabetes and even cancer. On top of, this information about the anti-inflammatory diet is provided.

The Fast & Fresh Anti-Inflammatory Cookbook is not a radical new 'fad' diet; it does not encourage you to live on bland and uninspiring foods; it does not recommend unrealistically small portion sizes; nor does it suggest that you need to stick to crazy 'one day off' and 'one day on' eating regimes. The recipes you will find in this cookbook do not require you to remain stuck at the stove for ages, preparing everyone else a lovely dinner, whilst you have to cook up an entirely separate bland and uninspiring dish for yourself.

Instead, the anti-inflammatory diet values fresh, inflammation reducing foods that are easy to prepare and delicious to eat! With this cookbook, you can continue to enjoy delicious meals with your loved one, family and friends, whilst at the same time reducing inflammation, symptoms and pain, and improving your overall health.

There are 150 scrumptious meal and drink ideas for you to try as well as useful information about the types of foods that should be avoided, and those you can continue to indulge in! The shopping lists will help you get started immediately and are designed to help you continue cooking the meals you love, without worrying whether the ingredients are going to flare up your symptoms and make you feel even worse.

Each of the recipes in this cookbook are made with easy to find fresh ingredients, are simple to prepare, and are either quick to bake, steam or sauté. We also include slow cooker recipes, giving you more time to get on with your busy life (or rest) whilst dinner's cooking!

Our philosophy is that if you take the time to understand which foods make you feel great and which flare up your symptoms, only cook with those that make you feel better, and stick to fresh and healthy options, then in time inflammation will start to reduce, and with that your symptoms.

This will not only help you to feel amazing but also get back on track with enjoying life rather than needlessly suffering.

Happy cooking and good luck on your anti-inflammatory journey!

The Lasselle Press Team

I

UNDERSTANDING INFLAMMATION

This chapter will address what inflammation, and the problems and symptoms that can be caused by chronic inflammation, in order to help you gain a better understanding of what may be going on in your body.

WHAT IS INFLAMMATION?

Inflammation is an auto-response system used by the body to remove toxins and repair damaged tissue as a result of illness or injury. It is an essential part of the body's healing process and is usually a positive and necessary reaction.

Let's take for example your knee becoming injured - when this happens, the body's immune system works to heal the knee itself. The knee may become swollen; chemicals such as histamine, bradykinin, and prostaglandins are released as a cell is damaged, and these chemicals will protect the body from further harm by causing the tissues to swell.

In turn, these chemicals are actually used to signal to the body that it needs help, and it needs help fast. The white blood cells recognize this recovery response, and attack any germs or bacteria present. These dead cells can then be seen in the form of puss, phlegm, or mucus.

This is usually always your body's way of protecting itself and is the natural response to injury. For many, the worst they might feel is a little bit of pain, which is called acute inflammation, and is a completely normal and healthy response.

But what if the inflammation doesn't go away?

What if the body's defence becomes its downfall?

That's when problems start. This prolonged inflammation is the type of inflammation discussed in this book: chronic inflammation. Symptoms and problems associated with chronic inflammation include joint damage, digestive issues, cardiovascular problems, and other diseases which we will go over in more detail later on.

Hopefully, this will help you understand chronic inflammation a little more, so that you can help yourself or someone you know deal with it in the best way possible.

CAUSES OF CHRONIC INFLAMMATION

Causes of chronic inflammation can range from lasting injuries, infections, toxin exposure or other autoimmune diseases.

SYMPTOMS OF ACUTE INFLAMMATION

Redness,
Pain in and around the affected area,
Increased body temperature,
Swelling.

These symptoms are usually experienced as a result of a viral infection or injury and will usually heal in due course without intervention.

SYMPTOMS OF CHRONIC INFLAMMATION

Chronic pain around the joints,
High blood pressure,
Redness and intense heat,
Intense swelling,
Tumours (in extreme cases),
Loss of function of the joint/affected area,
Food allergies,
Obesity,
Ulcers and skin problems such as dry skin, rashes, or puffy red eyes.

If you have any of these symptoms you should consult a doctor who can advise further, but there is a chance they could be a result of chronic inflammation.

INFLAMMATION AND DISEASE

Now let's take a look into what can happen to the body over time when suffering from chronic inflammation. Examples of illnesses and diseases that have been linked to chronic inflammation are as follows:

AUTOIMMUNE DISEASES: When our body's immune system is flawed and unable to tell the difference between our own cells and foreign cells, it will attack cells in our own body using auto-antibodies. As a result, the immune system does not work as it should do, and effectively works against the body. There are more than 80 known types of autoimmune disease. The common autoimmune diseases caused by inflammation are multiple sclerosis, Crohn's disease, diabetes, and celiac disease. Each disorder affects different parts of the body. Some of these (like celiac disease for example) are triggered by certain foods, in this case gluten, and you can help to alleviate the symptoms through dietary choices, which in turn will help reduce inflammation.

MULTIPLE SCLEROSIS: According to the US National Library of Medicine, MS is a severe auto-immune disease affecting the brain and spinal chord and damaging the protective sheaf around nerve cells. This damage is caused by inflammation and can occur around the brain, optic nerve or spinal chord. Whilst it is not known for certain what causes MS, it has been put down to a possible gene or virus defect, or even the environment.

DIABETES: Type 2 diabetes can be caused by a number of different factors, and inflammation can have a serious impact on diabetes because of insulin resistance in the body. Generally those with type 2 diabetes are advised to lose weight and reduce their intake of sugary and salty foods, but now that studies have linked inflammation with diabetes, clearly there is good reason to choose the anti-inflammatory diet in order to improve symptoms or even prevent them.

RHEUMATOID ARTHRITIS: This condition causes pain and inflammation of the joints. Most people take medications for arthritis but there is a link between the disease and diet, which is now recognized by many dietitians and doctors. Sometimes sugar, dairy, and processed foods can aggravate or cause the inflammation, and that's why so many people are suffering needlessly when simple dietary changes could make a real difference to their symptoms and pain.

ASTHMA: A chronic condition that can cause breathing problems. With asthma, air passages can become restricted due to inflammation which causes coughing, shortness of breath, and attacks in those who suffer severely.

OBESITY: There is evidence revealing a direct link between chronic inflammation and obesity: inflammation can cause insulin resistance, which in turn means the body stores more fat. Furthermore, chronic inflammation can even prevent healthy regulation of appetite. This is due to the signals that are sent to the brain that can cause resistance to Leptin (the hormone that tells your brain that you're full up). This, in turn, means you'll eat more, and thus gain weight.

ALLERGIES: Allergies are our body's reaction to certain proteins such as food, dust mites or pollen. When someone with an allergy is confronted with one of these proteins, allergens trigger the immune response, causing the body to go into self-defence mode. You may have experienced this in terms of sneezing, a blocked nose, or even swollen airways.

HEART DISEASE: It's the number one killer of people in the world today; inflammation of tissues can affect the heart, which can cause heart attacks, stroke and even heart failure. Sometimes the chemicals that are released to fight the problem can actually build up in the cells, thus restricting blood flow and making the threat to the heart even more severe.

CANCER: Research and studies have shown that chronic inflammation can actually predispose us to cancer.

This doesn't even begin to account for the other problems caused by or linked to inflammation such as Alzheimer's, Parkinson's, and depression. Simply put, chronic inflammation can cause horrible symptoms, diseases, and if not controlled, can get progressively worse.

The good news is that once you understand what's causing your symptoms or illness, you can try the anti-inflammatory cookbook to eat well, reduce inflammation and improve your health.

It is always recommended to consult your doctor or dietitian for advice and diagnosis before you change your diet, however the recipes featured in this book are all healthy, delicious and natural, therefore good for you and the rest of the family.

INFLAMMATION AND FOOD

As previously outlined, chronic inflammation can be caused by allergies or certain food types. You may have started to experience some of the previous symptoms after eating certain foods, as there is a direct correlation between our diets and inflammation in the body. That being said, you may not have linked certain food types with your inflammation and are unsure as to why you are experiencing your symptoms. Either way it is extremely important to consider our food choices when we are considering how to treat our pain.

For a healthy diet, our bodies need proteins, fats, carbohydrates, vitamins, and minerals, and anything we don't need is usually flushed out of the body through the digestive system. However, some toxins cause problems because they stay in the body when they shouldn't, thus triggering an immune response such as inflammation to try and get rid of these toxins. This will usually cause some kind of damage to the body.

Toxins sound like a scary word, but they're actually more prevalent than you might realize; there are over 100 toxins present in the body at any one time. These toxins range from chemicals commonly found in the pesticides sprayed on food, food dyes, and the most common toxin of all - preservatives. Preservatives are used in many food products, even some of the healthy whole grain and soy products that you wouldn't typically associate with toxins or chemicals. These preservatives are used to ensure a longer shelf life and are either natural (i.e. salt) or chemical. It's obviously the chemical preservatives that are most harmful but excess salt can too have adverse effects on our bodies.

The healthy body fights to get rid of these toxins and is usually successful in doing so, but with modern food and agriculture processes and an increase in packaged and ready-to-eat foods, our diets include so many toxins nowadays, that it's almost impossible for the body to eradicate them all.

Research and studies have revealed that a traditional Mediterranean diet with a high ratio of monounsaturated to saturated fats and polyunsaturated fats, plenty of fruit and vegetables, legumes and wholegrains is the best diet for anti-inflammatory effects. Overall the food you eat, and your doctor's advice and diagnosis, is key to feeling better, inside and out!

II

THE BENEFITS OF THE ANTI-INFLAMMATORY DIET

In this chapter, the benefits of the anti-inflammatory diet will be outlined, so that you can start eating the right foods for you, kick start inflammation reduction, and hopefully relieve the symptoms you've been experiencing as a result of chronic inflammation.

BENEFITS OF THE DIET

The anti-inflammatory diet helps reduce the amount of inflammation experienced in the body by removing the foods that typically cause inflammation. This should then help in reducing symptoms experienced and improving overall health. Further benefits of the anti-inflammatory diet are revealed below:

LESSEN THE RISK OF EXPERIENCING FURTHER ILLNESS OR DISEASE

Reducing inflammation will help you lessen your risk of experiencing one or more of the problems outlined in the previous chapter, including obesity and allergies. If you're at risk of heart disease, predisposed to diabetes, have high blood pressure, or you experience stiff and painful joints, then this diet is for you. Please always remember to consult a professional before making any changes to diet and lifestyle, especially when suffering from a pre-existing condition.

LOSE OR MAINTAIN WEIGHT IN A HEALTHY WAY

Likewise, if you're finding it hard to lose weight, you might not have considered inflammatory foods as the problem, as they aren't always associated with weight-gain. Maybe you've tried every single one of the popular diets going, and they just don't seem to work for you. The anti-inflammatory diet contains healthy and fresh ingredients that reduce inflammation and may also help you lose weight. Now, this isn't a fad diet and you probably won't drop a pant size in two weeks. But that's not the sole purpose of this change and there are many more benefits of losing weight gradually by changing your eating habits over the long term.

PREVENT FOOD ALLERGIES

As previously stated, the anti-inflammatory diet can also help with food allergies. Allergies can be problematic for many people, and if they're severe enough, they can be life threatening. Reducing inflammation can help minimize the severity or regularity of allergic reactions you experience.

GREAT FOR GLUTEN FREE

For many people who have a gluten allergy, this book can also help. A lot of the time people may not recognize gluten as a problem until they try a gluten-free diet. The anti-inflammatory nature of the foods used in this cookbook can actually help relieve the symptoms experienced by those who are intolerant to gluten.

IMPROVE YOUR SKIN

Anti-inflammatory foods can also greatly improve skin. Sometimes, inflammation can cause dry and ageing skin, redness, and even problems such as rosacea of the skin. This diet can help improve your skin's appearance, meaning you'll feel and look younger!

INCREASE YOUR ENERGY LEVELS

Moreover your energy will increase. Sometimes, we can feel a lack of energy when we consume inflammatory foods; it's not just sugars that sap our energy but processed foods as well. You are what you eat, as the old adage goes, and sometimes eating foods that cause tiredness and fatigue can be a major issue. These foods can also make you feel depressed. However, with the recipes in this cookbook, you can say goodbye to lethargy and depression by eating foods that give you energy and improve your quality of life.

REDUCE SYMPTOMS

Then there is the pain and soreness you may be experiencing. You shouldn't have to live with chronic pain and if you're not eating the right foods then your symptoms will certainly be worse than they need to be.

BE THE HAPPIEST AND HEALTHIEST VERSION OF YOURSELF

Making well-informed choices can change your life for the better. Try this diet and you will soon realize the potential that your body and mind have, and what you've been missing out on all this time. Don't let your health get in the way of feeling happy – eat well, live well and be well!

III

DIET STAPLES: WHAT TO KEEP IN YOUR KITCHEN

This chapter will go over the foods and ingredients that you can eat in order to help reduce inflammation. It will also outline those you should consider cutting out or limiting.

FOODS TO AVOID OR CUT DOWN:

Try keeping a food journal, logging what you've had to eat and drink each day, as well as a detailed description of any symptoms. That way you can start to track which foods seem to work well with your body and which do not. Try cutting out one food type at a time, to see what difference it makes.

HYDROGENATED OILS AND TRANS FATS:

These are found in many of the baked goods that we know and love. They are one of the main causes of inflammation in the body. You commonly find these in cookies, cakes and breads, and while they might taste good, they are best avoided because your body can't break them down properly.

SUGAR:

Now, not all sugars are bad, but we typically consume a diet loaded in sugar. Cut out synthetic sugars and try to reduce natural sugars such as honey to a minimum or a special treat!

SYNTHETIC SWEETENERS:

Sugar replacements such as aspartame, saccharin, sucralose and other chemicals found in diet sodas or sugar-free foods are toxic and inflammatory. Avoid synthetic sweeteners and replace with honey, maple syrup, or stevia if you need something sweet - all in moderation though!

MEAT:

Not necessarily bad for you, but can cause inflammation in some people. Commercial meat is what usually causes inflammation, as these animals are not typically fed on a healthy diet. If you do eat meat, go for grass-fed, hormone-free meat instead.

DAIRY:

Can cause sensitivity; reactions to the casein proteins in cow's milk is usually what causes inflammation. If you do experience discomfort after eating dairy, then it's best if you avoid it.

MERCURY:

Can be found in fish such as swordfish, and while having a little is okay, too much can be problematic. The UN Committee's recommended maximum intake is 1.6 micro-grams per kilogram of body weight per week. Check labels for the mercury levels in fish particularly.

GLUTEN:

Wheat can cause sensitivity in many people, and gluten can be inflammatory even for those who don't have the gluten allergy or celiac disease. You should also watch out for white flour, because it breaks down quickly, spiking your blood sugar levels and causing crashes and energy slumps soon after eating.

NIGHTSHADES:

Fruits and vegetables are encouraged on this diet, but nightshades can be a problem for some people. These include eggplants, potatoes, peppers, and tomatoes. They contain alkaloids, which can cause inflammation in those susceptible to them. There is some debate on this, as many have unique anti-inflammatory properties of their own. If you are unsure, eliminate one at a time from your diet and monitor in your food journal to see if this makes a difference. Alternatively, speak to a dietitian who can advise you personally.

OMEGA 6:

Causes high cholesterol and cardiovascular disease. The Western diet includes high levels of omega 6. Try to avoid seed and vegetable oils if you can, as these can cause a build up of omega 6 in the body. Opt for extra virgin olive or coconut oils instead.

PROCESSED FOODS:

Avoid these; it's not easy to do so at first because we are so reliant on them for quick and easy meals as part of a busy lifestyle. However, if you are able to avoid them, your symptoms should reduce dramatically.

ALCOHOL:

Make sure that you don't consume too much alcohol as it causes inflammation. Aim for 1-2 drinks a week maximum i.e. glass of wine/pint of beer/spirit.

FOODS TO BUY:

These are foods you should add to your shopping list. Replace the banned items with these and incorporate them into your daily diet right away!

WHOLE FRESH FOODS:

Enjoy meat, poultry, veggies, fruits and fish. Ideally, buy all of these organic, gluten-free, and grass-fed/free-range as these are foods in their natural states, without added chemicals and sugars. If budget is an issue, stick to fresh fruit and vegetables over tinned, and limit your intake of meat and poultry so that you have less but of a better quality.

FRUIT AND VEGETABLES:

These should be the staple of your diet as they include vital nutrients and help to keep you healthy with multiple benefits for skin, hair, and increased energy levels. Particularly choose:

TOMATOES: Rich in Vitamin C and cancer fighting but be careful as these are one of the nightshades. Keep a track of your foods in your journal to see what works for you. You can eat these raw or cooked.

LEAFY GREENS: Choose spinach and collards as their high Vitamin E content has been said to protect the body from the cells that cause inflammation. Their high calcium levels will also help supplement your diet if you do go dairy free.

STRAWBERRIES, RASPBERRIES AND BLUEBERRIES: The vibrant colors of fruits and vegetables is often a sign of their goodness.

GARLIC AND ONIONS: Both work at shutting down the process leading to inflammation.

BEETS: High in antioxidants and extremely anti-inflammatory, beets also help protect against heart disease and cancer.

MUSHROOMS: With so many varieties, mushrooms are an exciting and almost meaty addition to your meals. Great if you decide to cut out animal products completely. Mushrooms also have anti-inflammatory properties.

WHOLEGRAINS: Choose unrefined wholegrains such as oatmeal and quinoa (avoid white breads and flours). These should have no added sugars.

BEANS AND LEGUMES: You should eat these as part of a balanced diet as their high fiber content which will help detox waste from the body. These should be eaten in moderation – stick to 1 serving per day.

HEALTHY FATS:

Not all fat is bad. You should continue to include good fats, such as omega-3 fatty acids and unsaturated fats in your diet. Some of the fatty foods to choose a few times a week are:

HEALTHY FATTY FISHES HIGH IN OMEGA 3: SALMON, MACKEREL, TUNA, SARDINES – these should be eaten 2-3 times per week in order for the anti-inflammatory properties to work their magic! Fish oil supplements can also be taken and have beneficial effects, especially for rheumatoid arthritis sufferers.

OLIVE OIL/COCONUT OIL: Choose one or both of these as your main oils. Coconut oil is one of the healthiest fats out there and can be used for dressings, shallow frying and as part of your beauty regime!

ALMONDS AND WALNUTS: These nuts have a whole host of benefits including high antioxidant levels. Other nuts are also anti-inflammatory.

HERBS AND SPICES:

Use herbs and spices such as cloves, ginger, cumin, turmeric and rosemary (all of which are listed as the top 4 anti-inflammatory spices following a study by The University of Florida et al).

LOW-FAT DAIRY:

If you are keeping dairy in your diet, it is advised that you opt for low-fat or non-fat milk and yogurt options.

UNPROCESSED SOY PRODUCTS:

These are particularly beneficial for women in reducing inflammation because of the isoflavens (which are similar to the female hormone estrogen). Choose from soy milk, edamame beans and tofu. Also great for vegetarians.

You should start to throw away foods that aren't on the good list or perhaps donate them to a local homeless shelter or friend.

Keep any of the good foods that you have on the list and use this as a shopping list for your next trip to the store or market.

10 TIPS FOR THE ANTI-INFLAMMATORY DIET:

I AIM FOR AT LEAST 25 GRAMS OF FIBER EACH DAY

This is one of the most important tips as a high fiber diet will help to reduce inflammation. You should eat plenty of wholegrains, fruits and vegetables as your fiber sources.

II AIM FOR AT LEAST NINE SERVINGS OF FRUITS AND VEGETABLES EACH DAY.

You're probably wondering why we focus so much on fruit and veg in this diet. It's simple: they're anti-inflammatory foods and high in antioxidants. One serving = 1/2 cup of cooked vegetables or 1 cup of raw vegetables. Add spices to liven up the taste and increase antioxidant levels.

III AIM FOR AT LEAST FOUR SERVINGS OF BOTH ALLIUM AND CRUCIFEROUS VEGETABLES EACH WEEK.

Now, you're probably wondering what both of these are. Alliums are garlic, leeks, scallions and onions. Crucifers are vegetables such as cabbage, mustard greens, cauliflower, broccoli, and brussel sprouts. These all lower your risk of cancer, and help with inflammation. If you have four servings of these per week, the powerful antioxidants will be better able to eliminate toxins from your body.

IV LIMIT SATURATED FAT TO 10% OF YOUR DIET.

Only have red meat once a week and make sure to mix it with herbs, spices, and even unsweetened fruit juice to help with the toxic compounds that are released when cooking.

V OMEGA 3 FATTY ACIDS ARE YOUR FRIEND!

Omega-3 fatty acids can help to reduce inflammation in many different areas and help with many chronic diseases. Choose flax meal, beans, and walnuts as well as fish along with an omega 3 or fish oil supplement.

VI   EAT FISH AT LEAST THREE TIMES EACH WEEK

As previously explored, fish contains a host of nutrients, is generally low in calories in comparison to meat, and is an unsaturated 'good' fat. Oily fish as well as cold-water fish are great additions to the diet. If you're vegetarian, take an omega 3 tablet daily.

VII   CHOOSE THE RIGHT OILS

Fat is used to help with metabolic processes, and your cells need it to survive. Choose olive oil and coconut oil and buy organic where you can.

VIII   DON'T BE AFRAID TO SNACK

You can have a snack twice a day on this diet; choose healthy food types on the good food list. Try fruit, low fat Greek yogurt, raw fruit and vegetables, and nuts.

IX   AVOID PROCESSED FOODS

Processed foods and refined sugars are a big no-no on this diet. Foods high in fructose or sodium can also cause chronic inflammation to spike. You should try to avoid refined sugars when you can, and get rid of artificial sweeteners altogether.

X   CUT OUT TRANS FATS

In 2006, the FDA demanded that food companies identify trans fats on their nutrition labels. The protein in trans fats called a C –reactive protein can cause inflammation in the body. Not to mention, trans fats open the door to a host of diseases such as heart disease and diabetes. You should get into the habit of reading the labels on the foods you eat and checking for 'hydrogenated' or 'partially hydrogenated oils'. These should be avoided. These are often found in shortenings, some margarines, cookies, and crackers.

Hopefully these lists will help you get started stocking up your kitchen and cooking healthy meals that you can continue to enjoy both alone and with those around you, whilst being safe in the knowledge that you are eating the right foods to reduce your symptoms and become pain free.

IV

GETTING STARTED IN THE KITCHEN

This chapter provides an example 7 day meal plan, as well as cooking tips and kitchen equipment you'll need to help you get started with the anti-inflammatory diet.

7 DAY MEAL PLAN

Monday

Drink before Breakfast: Glass of water with Lemon

BREAKFAST: Tropical Coconut Delight

LUNCH: Middle Eastern Chicken Salad

DINNER: Nut Crusted Tilapia And Kale

Tuesday

Drink before breakfast: Glass of water with some lemon

BREAKFAST: Nutmeg & Cherry Breakfast Quinoa

LUNCH: Ginger, Carrot & Lime Soup

DINNER: Latino Black Bean Stew

Wednesday

Pre-Breakfast food: Glass of water with lemon

BREAKFAST: Gluten-Free Vanilla Crepes

LUNCH: Tasty Thai Broth

DINNER: Smoked Haddock & Pea Risotto

Thursday

Pre-Breakfast drink: Glass of water with lemon

BREAKFAST: Mini Fruit Muffins

LUNCH: Flavorsome Chicken Tagine

DINER: Sundried Tomato and Nut Pasta

Friday

Pre-breakfast drink: Glass of lemon water or lime water

BREAKFAST: Brilliant Buckwheat Breakfast

LUNCH: Tasty Thai Broth

DINNER: Italian Chicken & Zucchini Spaghetti

Saturday

Pre-Breakfast: Glass of water with
lemon

BREAKFAST: Fresh & Lean Sausage
Breakfast

LUNCH: Kipper & Celery Salad

DINNER: Pan Seared Salmon on
Baby Arugula

Sunday

Pre-breakfast: Glass of water with
lemon

BREAKFAST: Avocado Boats

LUNCH: Roasted Beets, Goats Cheese
& Egg Salad

DINNER: Chinese Orange-Spiced
Duck Breasts

Snacks

Feel free to have pick between 1 - 2
snacks per day between meals - See the
Sides & Snacks chapter for ideas!

COOKING TIPS

1. Grill, poach or bake meat, fish and poultry instead of frying. Use olive oil or coconut oil for sautéing.
2. Steam or boil vegetables instead of frying.
3. Use a slow cooker to free you up to do the things you enjoy!
4. Use spices and herbs to flavor foods instead of salts.
5. Cook in bulk and freeze leftover portions to take the load off your weekly cook.
6. Take the food lists from this book to the grocery store so that you can quickly remind yourself of the good foods to choose from as well as those to avoid.

KITCHEN EQUIPMENT

In order to help you get started on this diet, there are a few things that will be useful in order to be able to prepare the foods and meals in this cookbook:

- Blender/ food processor/mortar and pestle (optional)
- Crock pot, pans, skillet
- Steam basket/steamer/colander
- Oven dish, tray
- Potato masher
- Large mixing bowls
- Foil/cling film
- Tupperware boxes
- A 2 quart slow cooker for 2/4 quart slow cooker for families (optional)

EXERCISE :

Exercise is important and keeps you fit and healthy. However it is extremely important that you don't over-stress your body, as this can lead to inflammation. Walking, light jogs and exercise routines such as yoga and pilates are less strenuous but just as rewarding options. Consult your doctor for further guidance on this subject.

GETTING STARTED:

Now all that's left is to get started! We wish you all the best on your anti-inflammatory journey and hope that you will enjoy these recipes for a long time to come!

BREAKFAST

TROPICAL COCONUT DELIGHT

SERVES 2   PREP TIME: 2 MINUTES   COOK TIME: 10 MINUTES

A tropical fruity twist on your usual breakfast porridge.

---

2 CUPS WHOLEMEAL OATS (GF)

3 TSP RAW CACAO (OPTIONAL)

1/2 TSP STEVIA

3 CUPS COCONUT MILK

1 TSP COCONUT SHAVINGS

1 TBSP MILLED CHIA SEEDS

1/2 CUP MANGO/PINEAPPLE PIECES

---

1. In a pan mix the oats, cacao, stevia and coconut milk.
2. Heat on a medium heat and then simmer until the oats are fully cooked through (5-10 minutes).
3. Pour into your favorite breakfast bowl and sprinkle the coconut shavings, milled chia seeds, and fruit pieces on top.
4. Enjoy!

WARMING GINGERBREAD OATMEAL

SERVES 2   PREP TIME: 2 MINUTES   COOK TIME: 8 MINUTES

A winter warmer – delicious for breakfast or a supper-time treat by the fire!

---

2 CUPS STEEL CUT OR WHOLEMEAL OATS (GF)

3 CUPS WATER OR SOY MILK

1/2 TSP GROUND CINNAMON

1/2 TSP GROUND CLOVES

1/4 TSP GROUND GINGER

1/4 TSP GROUND ALLSPICE

1/4 TSP NUTMEG

1/4 TSP CARDAMOM

1 TSP HONEY TO TASTE

---

1. Mix the oats and water in a saucepan and gently heat on a medium heat for 5-8 minutes or until cooked through.
2. Whilst cooking stir in the spices.
3. When cooked and hot through, pour into your bowl.
4. Drizzle with a little honey and enjoy!

MINI FRUIT MUFFINS

SERVES APPROX. 6 MUFFINS   PREP TIME: 15 MINUTES   COOK TIME: 20 MINUTES

These delicious muffins are great for reducing inflammation.

---

1 CUP ALMOND MEAL

3 TSP STEVIA

2 TBSP CHOPPED CRYSTALLIZED GINGER

1 TBSP GROUND LINSEED MEAL

1/2 CUP BUCKWHEAT FLOUR

1/4 CUP BROWN RICE FLOUR

2 TBSP ORGANIC CORN FLOUR

2 TSP GLUTEN-FREE BAKING POWDER

1/2 TSP GROUND CINNAMON

1 CUP SLICED RHUBARB

1 APPLE, PEELED AND DICED

1 FREE RANGE EGG

1 TSP VANILLA EXTRACT

1/3 CUP ALMOND MILK

1/4 CUP EXTRA VIRGIN OLIVE OIL

---

1. Preheat oven to 350°f/180°c/Gas Mark 4.
2. Line a 6 hole muffin tin with coconut or olive oil using a baking brush or kitchen towel.
3. Add the almond meal, stevia, ginger, and the linseed meal into a mixing bowl.
4. Sieve the flours over the mix along with the baking powder and cinnamon and mix to combine.
5. Add the rhubarb and the apple into the mixture.
6. In a separate bowl, beat the egg, vanilla, milk, and oil until combined.
7. Fold the wet ingredients into the dry ingredients until a smooth batter is formed.
8. Pour batter into the muffin cases, leaving a 1 cm gap at the top so that the muffins can rise and then bake for 20 minutes or until risen and golden.
9. Remove and place on a cooling rack for 10 minutes before serving.

HANDY TIP: You can use a combination of any gluten free flours you can get your hands on as substitutes to the ones on this list.

BRILLIANT BUCKWHEAT BREAKFAST

SERVES 2   PREP TIME: 10 MINUTES   COOK TIME: 45 MINUTES

A tasty granola dish, perfect for breakfast!

---

1 CUP WHOLEMEAL OR STEEL CUT OATS (GF)	1/3 CUP OF PEELED AND FINELY CHOPPED APPLES
1/3 CUP BUCKWHEAT	1 TBSP COCONUT OIL
1/3 CUP SUNFLOWER SEEDS	2 CUPS WATER
1/3 CUP PUMPKIN SEEDS	1 TSP GINGER (FRESH AND GRATED)
1/3 CUP CHOPPED STRAWBERRIES OR RASPBERRIES	4 TBSP CACAO POWDER

---

1. Preheat the oven to 350°f/180°c/Gas Mark 4.
2. Mix the oats, buckwheat, and seeds in a bowl.
3. Add the fruit, coconut oil and water in a pan, cover and simmer for 10-15 minutes on a medium-high heat until the fruits are soft to touch. Then stir in the ginger.
4. Allow the fruit mixture to cool before adding to a blender with the cacao and blend until smooth.
5. Mix the fruits with the oat mixture.
6. Grease a baking tray with coconut oil and then spread the oat mixture on top using a knife or spatula to create a thin layer.
7. Bake for 45 minutes.
8. Stir the mixture every 15 minutes so it doesn't burn.
9. When crispy all over, remove the tray and allow to cool.
10. Serve as a crispy breakfast treat alongside low fat yogurt and fresh fruit if desired.

NUTMEG & CHERRY BREAKFAST QUINOA

SERVES 2   PREP TIME: 2 MINUTES   COOK TIME: 20 MINUTES

A complete protein, quinoa tastes brilliant sweet and savory, providing you with the energy you need. Cherries are a brilliant anti-inflammatory food.

1/2 CUP QUINOA

1/2 CUP UNSWEETENED FRESH CHERRIES

1 CUP WATER

1/4 TSP GROUND NUTMEG

1/2 TSP VANILLA EXTRACT

---

1. Into a pan combine all of the ingredients and cook over medium heat until bubbling.
2. Once bubbling, cover, lower the heat and simmer for 15 minutes or until the quinoa is soft and the liquid has been absorbed.
3. Pour into serving bowls and enjoy.

FRESH & LEAN SAUSAGE BREAKFAST

SERVES 4   PREP TIME: 8 MINUTES   COOK TIME: 15 - 20 MINUTES

Sausages are usually processed and should be avoided to fight inflammation, but this is a freshly cooked ground pork version which is delicious and healthy.

---

2 CUPS OF LEAN GROUND PORK

2 TSP FRESH CHOPPED SAGE LEAVES

1 TSP CHOPPED THYME

1 TSP GROUND BLACK PEPPER

1/4 TSP GROUND NUTMEG

1/4 TSP CAYENNE PEPPER

1/4 TSP CHOPPED ROSEMARY

1 TBSP EXTRA VIRGIN OLIVE OIL

---

1. Into a mixing bowl, combine all of the ingredients (except the oil).
2. Mix well until blended and then form 8 patties using the palms of your hands to shape.
3. Heat the oil in a skillet over a medium heat and cook the patties for 9 minutes one side and 9 on the other side until they're browned and cooked through.
4. Enjoy with a side of greens or a freshly boiled egg!

GLUTEN-FREE VANILLA CREPES

SERVES 2   PREP TIME: 5 MINUTES   COOK TIME: 10 MINUTES

These tasty crepes are great for anyone on the anti-inflammation diet or not - scrumptious and healthy!

---

2 FREE RANGE EGGS

1 TSP VANILLA

1/2 CUP NUT MILK OF YOUR CHOICE

1/2 CUP WATER

1 TSP MAPLE SYRUP

1 CUP GLUTEN-FREE ALL-PURPOSE FLOUR

2 TSP COCONUT OIL

---

1. Into a medium bowl add the eggs, vanilla, nut milk, water, and syrup together until combined.
2. Gradually, sieve the flour into the mix and whisk to combine to a smooth paste.
3. Take 1 tsp of the coconut oil and melt in a pan over a medium heat.
4. Add 1/2 crepe mixture, tilt and swirl the pan to form a round crepe shape.
5. Cook for about 2 minutes until the bottom is light brown and comes away from the pan with the spatula.
6. Flip and cook for a further 2 minutes.
7. Place crepe to one side, add 1 tsp coconut oil to the pan, and repeat with the rest of the mixture!
8. Enjoy with a squeeze of fresh lemon juice.

HANDY TIP: Keep an oven-proof plate in a warm oven so that you can keep the crepe nice and toasty whilst making the others - make extra batter and cook a load for the whole family!

MEDITERRANEAN VEGETABLE FRITTATA

SERVES 2   PREP TIME: 10 MINUTES   COOK TIME: 30 MINUTES

A zesty veggie treat, great on its own for breakfast or as a side with your favorite meal.

---

1 TSP COCONUT OR EXTRA VIRGIN OLIVE OIL

1 SWEET POTATO, PEELED AND SLICED USING POTATO SLICER OR SHARP KNIFE.

1 PEELED AND SLICED ZUCCHINI

4 FREE RANGE EGGS

2 TSP PARSLEY

1 TSP CRACKED BLACK PEPPER

---

1. Preheat broiler to a medium heat.
2. Heat the oil in a skillet under the broiler until hot.
3. Spread the potato slices across the skillet and broil for 10 minutes or until soft.
4. Add the zucchini to the skillet and cook for a further 5 minutes.
5. Meanwhile, whisk the eggs and parsley in a separate bowl, season to taste before pouring mixture over the veggies in the skillet.
6. Broil for 10 minutes under a low heat until golden brown and cooked through.
7. Remove and turn over onto a plate or serving board.
8. Cut the frittata into slices to serve.

AVOCADO BOAT BREAKFAST

SERVES 2   PREP TIME: 5 MINUTES   COOK TIME: 5 MINUTES

Poach the egg and float it in its own avocado boat; full of healthy fats and protein to start your day. Remember to eat one egg a maximum of twice a week.

---

1 RIPE AVOCADO

1 TBSP WHITE WINE VINEGAR

2 FREE RANGE EGGS

---

1. Place a large pan of water over a high heat and bring to the boil.
2. Once boiling add white wine vinegar (don't worry if you don't have it).
3. Lower the heat to a simmer and crack the eggs in.
4. Top tip: do it quickly and from a height to get a nice round shape.
5. Stir the water every now and then around the eggs to keep them moving and cook for 2 minutes for a very runny yolk; 2-4 minutes for a soft to firm yolk; and 5 for a hard yolk.
6. Whilst poaching, prepare your avocado by cutting through to the stone lengthways around the whole of the fruit.
7. Place one palm on each side of the avocado, twist, and it should come away into 2 halves.
8. Using your knife, carefully wedge it into the stone and pull to remove the stone. Alternatively, cut around the stone with the knife and use the sharp end to coax it out.
9. There will be a well in each half where the stone was.
10. Carefully scoop out your eggs with a ladle and place on top of each avocado half.
11. Season to taste and enjoy.

HANDY TIP: If you like your avocados grilled or broiled, turn the broiler to a medium heat and place each half with its poached egg underneath to broil for 5-6 minutes or until warm through.

CITRUS YOGURT BIRCHER

SERVES 2   PREP TIME: 2 MINUTES (REST OVERNIGHT IF POSSIBLE) COOK TIME: NA

This is a tasty fruity breakfast salad, high in antioxidants.

---

1 CUP OF WHOLEGRAIN STEEL CUT OATS (GF)

1 PINK GRAPEFRUIT PEELED AND SLICED (IF YOU CAN'T GET GRAPEFRUIT TRY MANGO)

2 ORANGES PEELED AND SLICED

16 OZ. LOW FAT GREEK YOGURT

HANDFUL OF FRESH CRANBERRIES OR CHERRIES FOR TOPPING

---

1. Mix the oats and fruit with the yogurt and allow to soak for as long as possible (overnight is best).
2. Serve and top with cranberries or cherries if desired – the oats should be nice and mushy and will have soaked up the flavors of the fruit.
3. Enjoy!

APRICOT & VANILLA PANCAKES

SERVES 2   PREP TIME: 4 MINUTES   COOK TIME: 5 MINUTES

These pancakes are so sweet and satisfying.

1/3 CUP BUCKWHEAT, BANANA OR ALMOND MEAL FLOUR

1 FREE RANGE EGGS

1/2 CUP ALMOND, HAZELNUT OR SOY MILK

1/2 TSP GLUTEN FREE BAKING POWDER

1 APRICOT PEELED AND CUBED

1 PEACH PEELED AND CUBED

1 TSP VANILLA EXTRACT

1 TBSP LOW FAT GREEK YOGURT TO SERVE

1 TSP COCONUT OIL

---

1. Preheat oven to its lowest setting.
2. Whisk all the ingredients (apart from the Greek yogurt and oil) until light and fluffy.
3. Place the batter to one side (you don't need to leave over night, they'll be just as scrummy cooked straight away).
4. Heat 1/4 coconut oil in a pan over a medium heat.
5. Pour 1/4 of the mixture into a pancake shape and cook for 1 minute.
6. Flip and repeat.
7. Stack on a plate and keep warm in the oven.
8. Repeat until you've used the rest of the mixture - adding a little coconut oil to the pan each time.
9. Serve with a dollop of Greek yogurt and extra fresh fruit if desired.

HANDY TIP: Make extra batter and keep in a sealed container in the fridge for 2-3 days.

CHIA BERRY SUPER FOOD

SERVES 2   PREP TIME: 5 MINUTES   COOK TIME: NA

This is a healthy and filling breakfast food that's so simple to make.

---

2 CUPS FRESH ORGANIC BLUEBERRIES

1 LARGE GREEN OR RED APPLE, PEELED AND SLICED

10 PITTED RAISINS

10 RASPBERRIES

2 TBSP CHIA SEEDS

1/2 CUP ALMONDS, RAW AND CHOPPED

1 TBSP CACAO POWDER

---

1. Add half the blueberries and apple to a sealed container.
2. Combine the rest of the blueberries with raisins and raspberries and blend until smooth (use a blender, food processor or hand held for this).
3. Add the blended mix to the apple and blueberries and pour in the chia seeds.
4. Top with the crushed almonds and a dusting of cacao powder to serve.
5. This can be kept in a sealed container in the fridge for up to 2-3 days.

MARVELLOUS MINI MEATLOAVES

SERVES 2   PREP TIME: 10 MINUTES   COOK TIME: 30 MINUTES

Tasty meaty treats.

1/2 CUP LEAN GROUND TURKEY	1 TBSP PAPRIKA
1/2 CUP GROUND CHICKEN	1/4 CUP COCONUT MILK
1 MINCED GARLIC CLOVE	SPRINKLE OF BLACK PEPPER
1/4 CUP CHIVES, FINELY CHOPPED	1 TSP COCONUT OIL
	] SPRINKLE OF CHOPPED PARSLEY

1. Preheat oven to 400°f/200°c/Gas Mark 6.
2. Mix turkey, chicken, garlic, chives, paprika, and coconut milk until the ingredients hold.
3. Season with black pepper to taste.
4. Line a 4 hole muffin tin with coconut oil and divide the mixture into each hole.
5. Bake in the oven for 30 minutes or until the meat is cooked through.
6. Sprinkle cooked meatloaves with parsley and serve alone or with side salad.

SWEETCORN & MUSHROOM FRITTATA

SERVES 4   PREP TIME: 5 MINUTES   COOK TIME: 20 MINUTES

A healthy snack great for any time of the day!

---

6 EGGS

1 CUP COCONUT MILK

1 TSP COCONUT OIL

1/2 CUP SWEETCORN (FRESH FROM THE COB OR FROZEN)

10 DICED MUSHROOMS

1 CUP ARUGULA

SPRINKLE OF PEPPER

---

1. Preheat the broiler to a medium heat.
2. Whisk the eggs and coconut milk in a bowl.
3. Heat the coconut oil in an oven proof (steel) frying pan over a medium heat.
4. Add sweet corn and mushrooms, and sauté for 5 minutes.
5. Spread the vegetables evenly across the pan.
6. Pour the egg mix over the vegetables and cook on a low heat for 7 minutes until the frittata starts to bubble.
7. Finish the frittata (in its pan) under the broiler for a further 5 minutes or until crispy on the top and cooked right through.
8. Serve with a side or arugula and season with black pepper.

BRUNCH

MIDDLE EASTERN CHICKEN SALAD

SERVES 2   PREP TIME: 10 MINUTES   COOK TIME: 20 MINUTES

Lightly spiced turmeric and cumin chicken.

FOR THE MARINADE:

1/2 CUP LOW FAT GREEK YOGURT

1 TBSP TURMERIC

1/4 TSP CUMIN

1/2 TSP GINGER, GRATED

1/2 TSP PAPRIKA

SPRINKLE OF GROUND PEPPER

1 TSP EXTRA VIRGIN OLIVE OIL

2 BONELESS, SKINLESS CHICKEN BREAST HALVES

FOR THE SALAD:

1/2 CUCUMBER, DICED

1 CUP WATERCRESS OR RAW SPINACH

1/2 CHOPPED ONION

1 TBSP OF CILANTRO, FRESHLY CHOPPED

2 TBSP FRESHLY SQUEEZED LEMON JUICE

---

1. Add the ingredients down to pepper with the yogurt into a bowl/Tupperware.
2. Marinate the chicken in the yogurt marinade for as long as possible.
3. Preheat broiler to a medium heat and grease a baking tray with olive oil.
4. Shake off the excess marinade from the chicken and then broil for 10 minutes (turning once half way).
5. Check the meat is thoroughly cooked and piping hot in the middle before removing from broiler and placing to one side.
6. Carefully slice chicken.
7. Meanwhile toss the salad ingredients together and drizzle with oil.
8. Serve sliced chicken on top of a bed of salad with lemon juice and cilantro over the top.
9. Enjoy.

PROTEIN SCOTCH EGGS

SERVES 2   PREP TIME: 10 MINUTES   COOK TIME: 25 MINUTES

These tasty protein breakfast bites are great for those on the go and won't flare up your symptoms.

16 OZ LEAN GROUND TURKEY

1/2 TSP BLACK PEPPER

1/2 TSP NUTMEG

1/2 TSP CINNAMON

1/2 TSP CLOVES

1/2 TSP DRIED TARRAGON

1/2 CUP FRESH PARSLEY, FINELY CHOPPED

1/2 TBSP DRIED CHIVES

1 CLOVE GARLIC, FINELY CHOPPED

4 FREE RANGE EGGS, BOILED AND PEELED

1. Preheat oven to 375°F/190°C/Gas Mark 5.
2. Cover a baking sheet with parchment paper.
3. In a large mixing bowl, combine the turkey with the pepper, nutmeg, cinnamon, cloves, tarragon, parsley, chives and garlic.
4. Mix well with your hands until thoroughly combined.
5. Divide the mixture into 4 circular shapes with the palms of your hands.
6. Flatten each one into a pancake shape using the backs of your hands or a rolling pin. You may need to wet your hands here to prevent sticking.
7. Wrap the meat pancake around 1 egg, until completely covered.
8. Bake in the oven for 25 minutes or until brown and crisp – check the meat is cooked through with a knife before serving.

CHINESE SPICED SALMON

SERVES 2   PREP TIME: 10 MINUTES   COOK TIME: 40 MINUTES

A fresh oriental staple with mustard - a superhero in the anti-inflammatory world.

---

2 SWEET POTATOES

1 TSP YELLOW MUSTARD SEEDS

2 5 OZ. SALMON FILLETS

1/2 CUP CHINESE BROCCOLI OR RAPINI

1 TSP HOT PREPARED CHINESE MUSTARD

---

1. Preheat oven to 400°f/200°c/Gas Mark 6.
2. Wrap the sweet potatoes in foil and roast in the oven for about 40 minutes or until tender.
3. Meanwhile, grind the mustard seeds in a pestle and mortar or blender and then rub over the salmon fillets.
4. Place the salmon fillets into the oven (wrapped in parchment paper for extra moisture) and cook for 12-15 minutes or until cooked through.
5. Meanwhile, boil a pan of water on a high heat and steam the broccoli over for 8-10 minutes, or until tender, before setting aside.
6. Remove sweet potatoes once cooked and allow to cool before scooping out the flesh and pureeing in a blender until smooth.
7. Stir the Chinese mustard into the sweet potato puree.
8. Serve the salmon fillets with a bed of broccoli and sweet potato puree on the side.
9. Enjoy.

CURRIED CHICKPEAS & YOGURT DIP

SERVES 2   PREP TIME: 10 MINUTES   COOK TIME: 15 MINUTES

Packed full of protein and anti-inflammatory spices.

---

1 TSP OLIVE OIL

1/2 ONION, PEELED AND CHOPPED

1 TSP GARLIC, PEELED AND MINCED

1 TBSP CURRY POWDER

1 TSP CUMIN

2 BEEF TOMATOES, CHOPPED (OPTIONAL)

1 CAN OF CHICKPEAS (DRIED IF YOU WISH BUT REMEMBER TO SOAK OVERNIGHT!)

1 TBSP CILANTRO

1/2 CUP LOW FAT GREEK YOGURT

1/2 CUCUMBER, DICED

1 SPRIG OF FRESH MINT, RIPPED INTO SMALL PIECES WITH YOUR FINGERS

1/2 FRESH LEMON

---

1. For the salad: heat the oil in a skillet over a medium-low heat.
2. Sweat the onion and garlic for 3-4 minutes, stirring until softened.
3. Add the curry powder and cumin to the onions and cook for about 2 minutes, whilst stirring as you smell the beautiful release of flavors!
4. Add in the tomatoes and cook over a medium high heat, stirring until the mix has thickened.
5. Add the chickpeas to the tomato mix before adding in the cilantro and cook for 5-6 minutes before covering and simmering on a low heat while you prepare the dressing.
6. Stir together the yogurt, cucumber, mint, and juice of ½ lemon.
7. Serve the chickpeas warm with a dollop of the yogurt dressing on top.
8. Enjoy.

SIRACHA STEAK WRAPS

SERVES 2   PREP TIME: 10 MINUTES   COOK TIME: 25 MINUTES

Succulent steak strips paired with crunchy pea shoots and lettuce.

---

2 TSP SESAME OIL

6 OZ LEAN SIRLOIN/RUMP STEAK

1 LARGE WHITE ONION, DICED

1 CLOVES OF GARLIC, DICED

2 TBSP SIRACHA

HANDFUL OF PEA SHOOTS OR CRESS

4 LARGE ICEBERG, ROMAINE, OR LETTUCE LEAVES FOR THE WRAPS

---

1. Heat 1 tsp oil in a skillet over a high heat, add the steak and cook for 6-10 minutes or according to package instructions.
2. Place to one side and allow to rest.
3. Wipe the pan clean.
4. Now heat 1 tsp oil and add the onions, cooking on a medium heat until browned for about 5 minutes.
5. Now add in the garlic and siracha to the onions and stir.
6. Slice the steak.
7. Remove from the heat and layer your steak slices and onion mix onto the center of each lettuce leaf.
8. Sprinkle over the pea shoots/cress before wrapping the lettuce around the beef like you would a fajita.
9. Serve your lettuce wraps warm and enjoy with your hands!

SPICY SHRIMP & ZUCCHINI NOODLES

SERVES 2   PREP TIME: 5 MINUTES   COOK TIME: 20 MINUTES

These shrimp noodles are fantastic in a jar and can be transported to work so easily –
say goodbye to your soggy sandwiches!

(FOR THE SEASONING)

1 TSP PAPRIKA

1/2 TSP CAYENNE PEPPER

DASH OF CHILLI FLAKES

12 JUMBO SHRIMP

1 TSP COCONUT OIL

3 CLOVES OF GARLIC, CRUSHED

1/2 WHITE ONION, FINELY SLICED

1 ZUCCHINI, SPIRALYZED OR CUT INTO THIN STRIPS

1 CARROT, SPIRALYZED OR CUT INTO THIN STRIPS

1/2 LIME

---

1. Combine the ingredients for the seasoning in a bowl and then add the shrimp to coat.
2. Heat the coconut oil and garlic in a pan on a medium to high heat, and then add the onion, sautéing for 2 minutes.
3. Add the dressed shrimp and cook until opaque.
4. Add the zucchini noodles for 3 minutes.
5. Add to a sealable glass jar and layer carrot slices on top.
6. Squeeze over the lime juice, cover and refrigerate for up to 2 days.
7. Enjoy right away or later on.

SPANISH LANGOUSTINE PAELLA

SERVES 2   PREP TIME: 15 MINUTES   COOK TIME: 40 MINUTES

A Mediterranean Masterpiece!

---

2 TBSP EXTRA VIRGIN OLIVE OIL

3 LARGE ORGANIC TOMATOES CUT INTO EIGHT PIECES (OPTIONAL)

A HANDFUL OF BLACK OLIVES

1 ZUCCHINI CUT INTO CUBES (ABOUT HALF CM THICK)

1 TBSP PAPRIKA

6OZ LANGOUSTINES, BUTTERFLIED

1 FRESH LEMON, CUT INTO QUARTERS

A HANDFUL OF COOKED FRESH PEAS

---

1. Heat oven to 325°f/170°c/Gas Mark 3.
2. Oil a baking tray and add the tomatoes, olives and zucchini.
3. Drizzle a little more olive oil over vegetables and sprinkle paprika over the top.
4. Toss to coat.
5. Oven bake for 30-40 minutes.
6. Whilst your vegetable mix is roasting, butterfly your langoustines: pull off the head and legs with your fingers and leave the tails on for presentation.
7. Score down the centre of each langoustine (do not slice in half) and then pull open on each side of the score to flatten.
8. Turn the oven up to 350°f/180°c/Gas Mark 4 and add langoustines to a roasting tray with an extra drizzle of olive oil.
9. Cook for 10 minutes, ensuring langoustines are piping hot before serving.
10. Mix the roasted vegetables with the cooked peas in a serving bowl.
11. Place the langoustines on top and serve with lemon chunks for squeezing.
12. Add pepper to taste.

HANDY TIP: Peppers can be added to the roasting tray if you find they don't flare up your symptoms: they have been noted for their anti-inflammatory vitamins, but are one of the nightshade vegetables so can be troublesome for some.

ORIENTAL CABBAGE & EGG BOWL

SERVES 2   PREP TIME: 5 MINUTES   COOK TIME: 15 MINUTES

These are so tasty and great for brunch or a healthy snack.

---

2 LARGE FREE RANGE EGGS

1 TBSP SESAME OIL

1 HEAD OF CABBAGE, SLICED

1 CARROT, SLICED

2 GREEN ONIONS, DICED

---

1. Boil a pan of water on a medium high heat and add the eggs to boil.
2. Cook for 5 minutes for a runny yolk or 7 minutes for a firmer yolk.
3. Meanwhile, melt the oil in a skillet over a medium heat and add the cabbage and carrot, sautéing until soft (5-6 minutes).
4. Add the green onions for the last minute.
5. Once eggs are done, run under cold water to remove the shell.
6. Serve the cabbage in serving bowls and top with peeled and halved boiled eggs .
7. Enjoy.

BURRITO BRUNCH

Marvelously Mexican!

---

2 CLOVES GARLIC

1 TBSP CHIPOTLE CHILI POWDER

1 TBSP APPLE CIDER VINEGAR

JUICE OF 1 LIME

2 TBSP EXTRA VIRGIN OLIVE OIL

2 TSP PEPPER

1 TSP PAPRIKA

1/2 TSP OREGANO

2 SKINLESS CHICKEN BREASTS

1 CUP QUINOA

JUICE OF 1 LIME

JUICE OF 1/2 LEMON

1/2 ICEBERG OR EQUIVALENT LETTUCE, (SHREDDED FOR SERVING)

2 TBSP CHOPPED CILANTRO

---

1. Take the garlic, chipotle powder, vinegar, lime juice, olive oil, pepper, paprika and oregano and blend in a blender or pestle and mortar.
2. Marinate the chicken in the marinade for as long as possible.
3. Heat the broiler to a medium-high heat.
4. Broil the chicken for 10-15 minutes (turning half way through) or until cooked through.
5. Remove and chop the chicken into cubes.
6. Meanwhile, boil a pan of water over a high heat and add the quinoa before covering and turning down the heat.
7. Allow to simmer for 15-20 minutes with the lid on.
8. Check its fully cooked (it will have soaked up most the water and turned translucent).
9. Serve quinoa with lime, lemon juices, chicken and shredded lettuce on top.
10. Sprinkle with cilantro and enjoy!

ITALIAN OPEN SANDWICH

SERVES 2 PREP TIME: 5 MINUTES COOK TIME: 30 MINUTES

A sandwich with a twist.

---

2 SKINLESS CHICKEN OR TURKEY BREASTS

1 CUP CHOPPED BASIL

1/2 CUP OF SPINACH

1/2 CUP PINE NUTS

1/2 TSP BALSAMIC VINEGAR

2 TBSP EXTRA VIRGIN OLIVE OIL

2 SLICES OF 100% WHOLEGRAIN BREAD (GF)

1 BEEF TOMATO, SLICED (OPTIONAL)

2 SLICES OF LOW FAT MOZZARELLA (LEAVE IF DAIRY FREE)

BLACK PEPPER TO TASTE

---

1. Preheat the oven to 375°F/190°C/Gas Mark 5.
2. Season chicken breasts with a little salt and pepper and wrap in baking/parchment paper.
3. Bake in the oven for 25-30 minutes or until cooked through.
4. Meanwhile, prepare the pesto by blending the basil, spinach and pine nuts in a blender or pestle and mortar with the balsamic vinegar and oil.
5. Add a little water to loosen the mixture if needed.
6. (Try using walnuts and/or almonds in the pesto if pine nuts are not available).
7. When chicken is thoroughly cooked through, toast the wholegrain bread under a broiler for a few minutes until golden.
8. Slice the chicken breasts.
9. Layer the bread with sliced tomato, mozzarella and chicken.
10. Sprinkle with pepper and serve with the pesto dressing to taste.
11. Enjoy.

LEMON CHICKEN & KOHLRABI SALAD

SERVES 2   PREP TIME: 10 MINUTES   COOK TIME: 10-15 MINUTES

Mouthwatering!

FOR THE MARINADE:

1 TBSP TURMERIC

1/4 TSP CUMIN

1/2 TSP GINGER, GRATED
SPRINKLE OF GROUND PEPPER

1 TSP EXTRA VIRGIN OLIVE OIL

2 BONELESS, SKINLESS CHICKEN BREAST
HALVES

FOR THE SALAD:

1/2 CUCUMBER, DICED

1 CUP WATERCRESS OR RAW SPINACH

1/2 CUP KOHLRABI, THINLY SLICED

2 TBSP. FRESHLY SQUEEZED LEMON JUICE

1 TBSP OF PARSLEY, FRESHLY CHOPPED

---

1. Combine the ingredients for the marinade before adding the chicken and covering.
2. If time allows, marinate for one hour up to overnight but don't worry if you need to cook right away!
3. Preheat broiler to a medium heat and grease a baking tray with olive oil. Shake off the excess marinade from the chicken and then broil for 10 minutes (turning once half way).
4. Check the meat is cooked and piping hot in the middle before removing from broiler and placing to one side.
5. Carefully slice chicken.
6. Meanwhile layer the salad onto serving plates and squeeze over the juice of your lemon.
7. Add finely chopped parsley to serve.
8. Enjoy.

QUINOA WITH CUCUMBER & MINT

SERVES 2 / PREP TIME: 10 MINUTES / COOK TIME: 15 MINUTES

Great for brunch or as a side dish.

---

1 CUP QUINOA

2 TBSP OLIVE OIL

1/2 ONION, PEELED AND CHOPPED

1 TSP GARLIC, PEELED AND MINCED

1 TBSP CURRY POWDER

1 TSP CUMIN

1/2 TSP TURMERIC

1 TBSP CILANTRO

1/2 CUCUMBER, DICED

1 SPRIG OF FRESH MINT, RIPPED INTO SMALL PIECES WITH YOUR FINGERS

1/2 FRESH LEMON

---

1. Add the quinoa to a pan of cold water (2 cups) over a high heat.
2. Allow to boil before covering, lowering the heat and simmering for 20 minutes or until the quinoa has soaked up the water.
3. Meanwhile, heat the oil in a skillet over a medium-low heat.
4. Sweat the onion and garlic for 3-4 minutes, stirring until softened.
5. Add the curry powder, cumin and turmeric to the onions and stir for about 2 minutes.
6. Add the cilantro.
7. For the dressing: mix the cucumber, mint, and juice of ½ lemon.
8. Mix the dressing through the quinoa and serve.
9. You can add low fat Greek yogurt to the dressing if your diet allows.
10. Enjoy.

SOUPS & BROTHS

GINGER, CARROT & LIME SOUP

SERVES 2   PREP TIME: 5 MINUTES   COOK TIME: 40 MINUTES

A real zingy soup – great for winter but can be served cooled in the summer too!

---

1 TBSP OLIVE OIL

1 TSP MUSTARD SEEDS, GROUND

1 TSP CORIANDER SEEDS, GROUND

1 TSP CURRY POWDER

1 TBSP GINGER, MINCED

4 CUPS CARROTS, THINLY SLICED

2 CUPS ONIONS, CHOPPED

ZEST AND JUICE OF 1 LIME

4 CUPS LOW-SALT VEGETABLE BROTH

BLACK PEPPER FOR TASTE

---

1. In a large pan over a medium heat, add the oil, the seeds and curry powder for 1 minute.
2. Add the ginger and then cook for another minute.
3. Now add in the carrots, onions, and the lime zest, cooking for at least 5 minutes or until the vegetables are soft.
4. Add the broth and bring to the boil before turning down the heat to medium and allowing to simmer for 30 minutes.
5. Allow to cool.
6. Put the mixture in a food processor and blend until smooth.
7. Serve with lime juice and black pepper.
8. Enjoy.

ASIAN SQUASH & SHITAKE SOUP

SERVES 2   PREP TIME: 10 MINUTES   COOK TIME: 45 MINUTES

Chinese mushrooms can be enjoyed endlessly on the anti-inflammatory diet and make a delicious soup.

---

15 DRIED SHITAKE MUSHROOMS, SOAKED IN WATER

3 CUPS LOW SALT VEGETABLE BROTH

1/2 BUTTER NUT SQUASH, PEELED AND CUBED

1 TBSP SESAME OIL

1 ONION, QUARTERED AND SLICED INTO RINGS

1 LARGE GARLIC CLOVE, CHOPPED

4 STEMS OF PAK CHOY OR EQUIVALENT

1 SPRIG OF THYME OR 1 TBSP. DRIED THYME

1 TSP TABASCO SAUCE (OPTIONAL)

---

1. Heat sesame oil in a large pan on a medium high heat before sweating the onions and garlic.
2. Add the vegetable stock and bring to a boil over a high heat before adding the squash.
3. Turn down heat and allow to simmer for 25-30 minutes.
4. Soak the mushrooms in the water if not already done, and then press out the liquid and add to the stock into the pot.
5. Use the mushroom water in the stock for extra taste.
6. Add the rest of the ingredients except for the greens and allow to simmer for a further 15 minutes or until the squash is tender.
7. Add in the chopped greens and let them wilt before serving. Serve with the tabasco sauce if you like it spicy.

SPICED RED PEPPER & TOMATO SOUP

SERVES 2   PREP TIME: 2 MINUTES   COOK TIME: 30 MINUTES

Hot and Spicy!

---

2 RED BELL PEPPERS, SLICED IN HALF

4 BEEF TOMATOES

1 SWEET ONION, CHOPPED

1 GARLIC CLOVE, CHOPPED

2 HABANERO CHILIS WITH THE STEMS REMOVED AND CHOPPED

2 TBSP OF EXTRA VIRGIN OLIVE OIL

3 CUPS HOMEMADE CHICKEN/VEGETABLE BROTH

---

1. Preheat the broiler to a medium-high heat and broil the bell peppers on an oven tray.
2. Turn half way through cooking time and cook until the skins are blackened (10 minutes).
3. Meanwhile, bring a pan of water to the boil over a high heat.
4. Cut a small x at the bottom of each tomato using a sharp knife.
5. Blanch the tomatoes in simmering water for about 20 seconds.
6. Remove and plunge into ice cold water.
7. Peel and chop tomatoes, reserving the juices.
8. Transfer peppers once cooked to a separate dish and cover.
9. Saute the onion, garlic, chilis and 2 tbsp of oil in a skillet over a medium-high heat, stirring until golden for 8-10 minutes.
10. Add the tomatoes with their juices, the peppers and broth to the onions.
11. Cover and simmer for 10-15 minutes or until heated through.
12. Allow to cool slightly before blending.
13. Enjoy!

HANDY TIP: avoid this one if you can't tolerate nightshades.

TASTY THAI BROTH

SERVES 2   PREP TIME: 5 MINUTES   COOK TIME: 25 MINUTES

The taste of Thailand can easily be conjured with this fresh and zesty dish.

---

1 TBSP CORIANDER SEEDS

1 RED CHILI, FINELY CHOPPED

A HANDFUL OF FRESH BASIL LEAVES

2 TBSP OLIVE OIL

1 WHITE ONION, CHOPPED

1 GARLIC CLOVE, MINCED

1 THUMB SIZE PIECE OF GINGER, MINCED

1/2 CUP OF COCONUT MILK

1/2 CUP OF HOMEMADE CHICKEN BROTH

2 SKINLESS COD FILLETS

1 PAK CHOY (LEAVES PULLED OFF SEPARATELY BUT NOT SLICED)

2 HANDFULS BABY SPINACH LEAVES

1 FRESH LIME

1/4 CUP SCALLIONS, CHOPPED

---

1. Crush the coriander seeds, chili and basil in a blender or pestle and mortar.
2. Mix in 1 tbsp of olive oil until a paste is formed.
3. Heat a large pan/wok with sesame oil on a high heat.
4. Fry the onions, garlic and ginger for 5-6 minutes until soft but not crispy or browned.
5. Add the spice paste with the coconut milk into the pan and stir.
6. Slowly add the broth.
7. Now add your fish fillets and allow to simmer in the broth for 10-15 minutes or until cooked through.
8. Add the pak choy and spinach 2-3 minutes before the end of the cooking time.
9. Serve with the fresh lime wedges.
10. Serve hot with scallions sprinkled over the top.
11. Enjoy.

MOROCCAN SPICED LENTIL SOUP

SERVES 2   PREP TIME: 5 MINUTES   COOK TIME: 40 MINUTES

Lentils are rich in folic acid and can be enjoyed up to twice a day. They are delicious in this Moroccan inspired soup.

1 TBSP EXTRA VIRGIN OLIVE OIL	1/2 TSP GROUND TURMERIC
1 YELLOW ONION, DICED	1 CAN CHOPPED TOMATOES
1 CARROT, DICED	2 TBSP LOW FAT GREEK YOGURT
1 CLOVES OF MINCED GARLIC, DICED	1 CUP DRIED YELLOW LENTILS, SOAKED OVERNIGHT/CANNED LENTILS
1 TSP GROUND CUMIN	
1/2 TSP GROUND GINGER	2 CUPS OF LOW SALT VEGETABLE BROTH HOMEMADE CHICKEN BROTH
1/2 TSP RED CHILI FLAKES	1 LEMON

1. In a large pan, heat the oil over a medium-high heat.
2. Sauté the onion and carrot for 5-6 minutes , until softened and starting to brown.
3. Add the garlic, cumin, ginger, chili flakes and turmeric, stirring for 2 minutes.
4. Add the tomatoes, scraping any brown bits from the bottom of the pan and cooking until the liquid is reduced (15-20 minutes).
5. Add the lentils and stock and turn the heat up to reach a boil before lowering heat, covering and simmering for 10 minutes.
6. Allow to cool slightly before blending until smooth. Alternatively, serve as a chunky rustic soup.
7. Serve with a wedge of lemon on the side and a dollop of Greek yogurt.
8. Enjoy.

FLAVORSOME VEGETARIAN TAGINE

SERVES 2   PREP TIME: 10 MINUTES   COOK TIME: 35 MINUTES

A vegetarian take on a Moroccan classic.

---

1 TBSP COCONUT OIL	1 SWEET POTATO, PEELED & DICED
1 ONION, DICED	4 BABY CARROTS, PEELED & DICED
1 PARSNIP, PEELED AND DICED	4 CUPS LOW-SALT VEGETABLE BROTH
2 CLOVES OF GARLIC	2 CUPS KALE LEAVES
1 TSP GROUND CUMIN	2 TBSP LEMON JUICE
1/2 TSP GROUND GINGER	1/4 CUP CILANTRO, ROUGHLY CHOPPED
1/2 TSP GROUND CINNAMON	HANDFUL OF TOASTED ALMONDS
3 TBSP TOMATO PASTE	
1/4 TSP CAYENNE PEPPER	

---

1. Heat the oil in a large pan over a medium-high heat before sautéing the onion until soft.
2. Add the parsnip for 10 minutes or until golden brown.
3. Add the garlic, cumin, ginger, cinnamon, tomato paste, and cayenne pepper.
4. Cook for about 2 minutes until the lovely scents reach your nose.
5. Fold in the sweet potatoes, carrots, and broth and then bring to a boil.
6. Turn heat down and simmer for 20 minutes.
7. Add in the kale and lemon juice in the last 10 minutes and cook until the leaves are slightly wilted.
8. Garnish with the cilantro and the nuts to serve.
9. Enjoy.

HANDY TIP: If toasting your own almonds, simply heat a dry skillet over a medium-high heat and add the almonds until they start to toast but not burn (about 4 minutes).

WINTER WARMING CHUNKY CHICKEN SOUP

SERVES 4   PREP TIME: 10 MINUTES   COOK TIME: 40 MINUTES

Nostalgic and homemade – beats inflammation and warms the soul!

---

1 WHOLE FREE RANGE CHICKEN (NO GIBLETS), COOKED

1 BAY LEAF

5 CUPS OF HOMEMADE CHICKEN BROTH/WATER

1 ONION, CHOPPED

2 STALKS OF CELERY, SLICED

3 CARROTS, CHOPPED AND PEELED

2 PARSNIPS, CHOPPED AND PEELED

SPRINKLE OF PEPPER TO SEASON

---

1. Add all of the ingredients minus the pepper into a large pot and bring to the boil over a high heat.
2. Once boiling, lower the heat to medium, cover and simmer for 30 minutes, or until the chicken is piping hot throughout.
3. Remove the chicken and place on a chopping board.
4. Slice as much meat as you can from the chicken and remove the skin and bones.
5. Add it back into the pot, stir, and either serve right away as a chunky soup or allow to cool before blending into a smooth soup.
6. Add black pepper to season and serve alone or with gluten free wholegrain bread.
7. (Quinoa tastes delicious with this too – just pop it into the soup 20 minutes before the end and it will soak up all the delicious chicken flavors).

HANDY TIP: If you have leftovers, strain and keep in a sealed container as chicken broth. You can keep this for 2-3 days in the fridge or 3-4 weeks in the freezer.

CURRIED LENTIL & SPINACH STEW

SERVES 2   PREP TIME: 5 MINUTES   COOK TIME: 30 MINUTES

A hearty and wholesome stew made with the flavors of India.

1 TBSP EXTRA-VIRGIN OLIVE OIL	TABLE BROTH
1 ONION, CHOPPED	1 CUP RED LENTILS, SOAKED OVERNIGHT OR CANNED
2 GARLIC CLOVES, MINCED	2 CUPS BUTTER NUT SQUASH, COOKED PEELED AND CHOPPED
1 TBSP CURRY POWDER	
1 TSP GROUND GINGER	1 CUP SPINACH
1 CUP HOMEMADE CHICKEN OR VEGE-	1 TBSP CILANTRO, FINELY CHOPPED

1. Into a large pot, add the oil, chopped onion and minced garlic, sautéing for 5 minutes on low heat.
2. Add the curry powder and ginger to the onions and cook for 5 minutes.
3. Add the broth and bring to a boil on a high heat.
4. Stir in the lentils, squash and spinach, reduce heat and simmer for a further 20 minutes.
5. Allow to cool before blending or serve as a chunky soup.
6. Season with pepper to taste and serve with fresh cilantro.
7. Enjoy.

HOMEMADE VEGETABLE BROTH

SERVES 2   PREP TIME: 10 MINUTES   COOK TIME: 35 MINUTES

A simple stock recipe for use in many of the recipes in this cookbook.

1 TBSP EXTRA VIRGIN OLIVE OIL	1 BAY LEAF
2 ONIONS, ROUGHLY CHOPPED	1 TBSP THYME
3 CARROTS, ROUGHLY CHOPPED	1 TBSP PARSLEY
3 CELERY STALKS, ROUGHLY CHOPPED	1 TSP BLACK PEPPERCORNS
1 GARLIC CLOVE, MINCED	

1. Chop your vegetables into large chunks (quarters at the smallest).
2. Leave the skins on as they add to the taste and the nutrients - add to the pan.
3. Heat the oil in a large pot over a medium heat and add the vegetables, garlic, herbs and peppercorns, cooking for 5 minutes.
4. Fill up the pot with boiling water.
5. Turn up the heat and bring to the boil - allow to simmer for 25 minutes.
6. Strain stock and use immediately or allow to cool and refrigerate for 2-3 days or freeze for 3-4 weeks in a sealed container.

HANDY TIP: You can use this broth for many of the recipes in this cookbook.

HOMEMADE HEALTHY CHICKEN BROTH

SERVES 2   PREP TIME: 10 MINUTES   COOK TIME: 4 HOURS

This homemade chicken broth is far healthier than shop bought.

1 WHOLE ROASTING CHICKEN {AROUND 4-5LBS}	**3 STALKS OF CELERY, SOAKED IN WARM WATER**
3 CARROTS, SOAKED IN WARM WATER	**1 TBSP EACH DRIED ROSEMARY, THYME, PEPPER, TURMERIC**
2 MEDIUM ONIONS	**1 TBSP WHITE WINE VINEGAR**
4 GARLIC CLOVES, CRUSHED	**11-12 CUPS WATER**
2 BAY LEAVES	

1. Rinse off your chicken and place in a large saucepan or soup pan (remove giblets but don't waste them; add them in to your stock pot!)
2. Chop your vegetables into large chunks (quarters at the smallest).
3. Leave the skins on as they add to the taste and the nutrients - add to the pan.
4. Add the rest of the ingredients to the pan.
5. Fill your pan with water so that the chicken and vegetables arc completely covered.
6. Turn stove on high and bring to boiling point before reducing the heat, covering and simmering for 3-4 hours.
7. Check at intervals and top up with water if the ingredients become uncovered.
8. Take off the heat and carefully remove the chicken, placing to one side.
9. You now need to strain the liquid from the stockpot into another bowl using a sieve to get rid of all the lumpy bits.
10. Leave the stock and chicken to cool.
11. Once cool, tear or cut the meat from the bones and save for a chicken soup, sandwich or cold meat brunch!
12. Once the stock has cooled to room temperature, add to a sealed container and keep in the fridge for 2-3 days or the freezer for 2-3 weeks.

HANDY TIP: You can use this broth for many of the recipes in this cookbook.

SMOOTHIES AND DRINKS

GINGERY GREEN ICED-TEA

SERVES 1   PREP TIME: 5 MINUTES   COOK TIME: NA

A refreshing iced-tea with anti-inflammatory properties.

---

2 CUPS CONCENTRATED GREEN OR MACHA TEA, SERVED HOT

1/4 CUP CRYSTALYZED GINGER, CHOPPED INTO FINE PIECES

1 WEDGE OF LEMON

1 SPRIG OF FRESH MINT

---

1. Mix the tea with the ginger in a glass teapot or serving mug and then cover and chill for as long as time permits.
2. Strain and pour into serving glasses over ice if you wish.
3. Garnish with a wedge of lemon and a sprig of fresh mint to serve.
4. Enjoy.

MULTI-VITAMIN SMOOTHIE

SERVES 2   PREP TIME: 5 MINUTES   COOK TIME: NA

This delectable smoothie is full of powerful antioxidants.

1/4 CUP RED OR WHITE GRAPES

1/4 CUP SLICED FROZEN OR FRESH PEACHES

1/4 CUP CHOPPED CABBAGE

1 CARROT, PEELED AND SLICED

1/2 CUP ICE CUBES

2 CUPS WATER

1 SPRIG OF FRESH MINT

---

1. Toss all of the ingredients in a blender or juicer until smooth.
2. Serve immediately in a tall glass with fresh mint to garnish.

BANANA & APPLE SMOOTHIE

SERVES 1   PREP TIME: 5 MINUTES   COOK TIME: NA

A filling breakfast or snack to fuel you until your next meal.

1 BANANA	2 CUPS FILTERED WATER
1 APPLE, CORED AND PEELED	1 TBSP STEVIA
2 TBSP FLAXSEED OIL	1 CUP LOW FAT COCONUT MILK
2 TBSP WHOLE OAT BRAN	1 CUP OF SPINACH OR EQUIVALENT GREEN OF YOUR CHOICE

1. In a food processor, add all of the ingredients except for the greens, processing until smooth.
2. Mix in the greens and then blend until smooth.
3. Serve over ice and enjoy.

BLUEBERRY AND SPINACH SHAKE

SERVES 1   PREP TIME: 2 MINUTES   COOK TIME: NA

Packed with antioxidants and iron.

---

1 CUP OF LOW FAT GREEK YOGURT
(OPTIONAL)

1 CUP ORGANIC BLUEBERRIES (OR
WASHED IF NON-ORGANIC)

1/2 CUP SPINACH

ICE CUBES TO DESIRED CONCENTRATION

---

1. Add ingredients together in a blender until smooth and then serve in a tall glass.
2. Sprinkle over a few fresh berries on top if you wish!

ANTIOXIDANT SMOOTHIE

SERVES 1   PREP TIME: 2 MINUTES   COOK TIME: NA

Great for boosting brain power and reducing inflammation at the same time.

---

1 CUP FROZEN BLUEBERRIES

1/2 BANANA

1/2 CUP CUCUMBER, CHOPPED

1 TBSP FLAX SEEDS

1 CUP COCONUT WATER

---

1. Take all of the ingredients and blend until smooth.
2. You can add ice cubes at this point if you want it chilled.
3. Serve and enjoy.

SYMPTOM SOOTHING SMOOTHIE

SERVES 1   PREP TIME: 2 MINUTES   COOK TIME: NA

An immediate pain relief for when your symptoms flare up.

---

1 STALK CELERY, CHOPPED

1 CUP CUCUMBER, CHOPPED

1/2 CUP PINEAPPLE, CHOPPED

1/2 LEMON, ZEST JUICE

1 CUP COCONUT WATER

1 APPLE, CHOPPED

---

1. Take all of the ingredients (minus the lemon zest) and blend until smooth.
2. You can add ice cubes at this point if you want it chilled.
3. Serve with a sprinkling of lemon zest.

WONDERFUL WATERMELON DRINK

SERVES 1   PREP TIME: 2 MINUTES   COOK TIME: NA

This is a great fruit juice packed with an array of vitamins.

---

1 CUP WATERMELON CHUNKS

2 CUPS FROZEN MIXED BERRIES

1 CUP COCONUT WATER

2 TBSP CHIA SEEDS

1/2 CUP OF TART CHERRIES

---

1. Blend ingredients in a blender or juicer until smooth.
2. Serve immediately and enjoy!

SWEET & SAVOURY SMOOTHIE

SERVES 1   PREP TIME: 10 MINUTES   COOK TIME: NA

The spices used in this smoothie make it fantastic for anti-inflammatory purposes but also a more savory drink between meals.

---

2 CUPS CARROTS, PEELED AND SLICED

2 CUPS FILTERED WATER.

1 APPLE, PEELED AND SLICED

1 BANANA, PEELED AND SLICED

1 CUP FRESH PINEAPPLE, PEELED AND SLICED

1/2 TBSP GINGER, GRATED

1/4 TSP GROUND TURMERIC

1 TBSP LEMON JUICE

1 CUP ALMOND OR SOY MILK

---

1. Blend carrots and water until smooth.
2. Pour into a Mason jar or sealable container, cover and place in fridge.
3. Once done, add the rest of the smoothie ingredients to a blender or juicer until smooth.
4. Add the carrot juice in at the end, blending thoroughly.
5. Serve with or without ice and enjoy.

BLACKBERRY & GINGER MILKSHAKE

SERVES 1   PREP TIME: 2 MINUTES   COOK TIME: NA

An unusual yet sensational blend of flavors!

---

1 THUMB SIZED PIECE OF GINGER, GRATED

2 CUPS BLACKBERRIES, WASHED

2 CUPS CHOPPED PEACHES

2 CUPS ALMOND MILK

---

1. Add all the ingredients to a blender or juicer until smooth.
2. Serve with a scattering of fresh blackberries and enjoy!

ALMOND & TURMERIC CHAI TEA

SERVES 4   PREP TIME: 2 MINUTES   COOK TIME: 2 MINUTES

A timeless healer, turmeric is used for its anti-inflammatory properties and makes a delicious chai!

3 TBSP TURMERIC	1 TSP CAYENNE PEPPER
4 TSP CINNAMON	4 TSP CHAI TEA POWDER
1/8 TSP GROUND CLOVES	4 CUPS BOILING WATER
1 TSP GROUND CARDAMOM	HONEY TO TASTE
1 TSP GROUND GINGER	1 CUP ALMOND MILK

1. Combine all of the ingredients excluding the milk and honey in a glass container, mix well and then seal.
2. Pour boiling water into 2 tbsp of the tea mix (use a tea strainer to serve).
3. You can then add almond milk and honey to taste.
4. Save the tea mix in a sealed container, storing in a dry place for future chais!
5. Enjoy.

HOMEMADE APPLE TEA

SERVES 4   PREP TIME: OVERNIGHT   COOK TIME: NA

If you like something a little more sweet, this apple-infusion is perfect for you.

---

4 CUPS BOILING WATER

4 TBSP FRESH GREEN TEA LEAVES

2 APPLES, PEELED AND SLICED.

1 TSP CINNAMON

A SPRIG OF FRESH MINT

---

1. Into a teapot, pour boiling water over the tea leaves through a tea strainer, allowing to steep for 5 minutes.
2. Add the apple slices and cinnamon to the boiling water and transfer into a sealable container.
3. Chill overnight to allow apple to infuse before serving.
4. Garnish with fresh mint to serve over ice.
5. Enjoy.

FRESH CRANBERRY & LIME JUICE

SERVES 4   PREP TIME: 5 MINUTES   COOK TIME: NA

An anti-inflammatory blend for your juicer.

---

4 CUPS CRANBERRIES

2 LIMES, JUICED

1/2 CUP SPINACH

1/2 CUP OF MIXED BERRIES (FROZEN ARE FINE)

4 CUP WATER

---

1. Mix all the ingredients with water in a juicer until smooth (you may need to do this in 2 batches).
2. Serve immediately over ice.
3. Enjoy!

FRESH TROPICAL JUICE

SERVES 4   PREP TIME: 5 MINUTES   COOK TIME: NA

A Caribbean treat, helping you fight symptoms and continue enjoying sweet drinks.

---

1 WHOLE FRESH PINEAPPLE, PEELED AND CUT INTO CHUNKS.

1/2 CAN LOW FAT COCONUT MILK

1 CUP WATER

---

1. Add all ingredients to a juicer and blend until smooth.
2. Serve over ice and enjoy.

MIXED FRUIT & NUT MILKSHAKE

SERVES 2   PREP TIME: 5 MINUTES   COOK TIME: NA

This smoothie not only contains the antioxidants found in fruit, but has protein from the nuts too.

1/2 GRAPEFRUIT, PEELED AND CHOPPED

2 TBSP CHOPPED ALMONDS

1/2 INCH PIECE OF GINGER, MINCED

JUICE OF 1 ORANGE

1 TBSP HONEY

1/2 CUP ALMOND MILK

12 STRAWBERRIES

1. Put everything but the strawberries in a blender until smooth.
2. Add the strawberries and blend until smooth.
3. Serve in a tall glasses and enjoy.

SUPER STRAWBERRY SMOOTHIE

SERVES 2   PREP TIME: 5 MINUTES   COOK TIME: 30 MINUTES

A sweet treat to be enjoyed without any guilt!

1 STALK OF CELERY, CHOPPED	1 CUP STRAWBERRIES
1/2 CUP OF KALE	1 LIME WEDGE
1/2 CUP OF SPINACH	1 CUP COCONUT WATER

1. Take all of the ingredients and blend until smooth.
2. Serve over ice and enjoy.

PEACH ICED TEA

SERVES 2   PREP TIME: 5 MINUTES   COOK TIME: NA

A perfect thirst-quencher.

---

2 CUPS CONCENTRATED GREEN OR MACHA TEA, SERVED HOT

1 PEACH, PEELED AND SLICED

2 WEDGES OF LEMON

---

1. Get a glass container, mix the tea with the peach slices, and then cover and chill for as long as time permits.
2. Strain and pour into serving glasses (over ice if you wish).
3. Garnish with a wedge of lemon to serve.

BEEF AND PORK MAIN DISHES

HERBY CHUCK ROAST & SCRUMMY VEG

SERVES 4   PREP TIME: 10 MINUTES   COOK TIME: 7 HOURS IN CROCK POT

This is an awesome meal to be shared with the family!

---

16 OZ OF LEAN CHUCK ROAST

1 TSP PEPPER

SEASONING:

1 TBSP CAYENNE PEPPER

2 TBSP DRIED/FRESH ROSEMARY

2 ONIONS CUT, PEELED AND QUARTERED

8 BABY CARROTS, PEELED AND QUARTERED

1 STALK OF CELERY, SLICED

1 BAY LEAF

10 CUPS WATER

1 CAULIFLOWER, CUT INTO FLORETS

---

1. Use a sharp knife to trim any remaining fat from the chuck roast.
2. Season the meat with the herbs and spices.
3. Put the onions, carrots, and celery into the crock pot/slow cooker, then the meat, and finally add the bay leaf and water.
4. Cook on low for about 5-7 hours or until the meat is tender.
5. You can then add the cauliflower for the last 15 minutes or until cooked through.
6. Serve hot and enjoy with your choice of quinoa or sweet potato.

FAST AND FRESH LEAN BEEF BURGERS

SERVES 2   PREP TIME: 5 MINUTES   COOK TIME: 25 MINUTES

Yes you can still enjoy a burger from time to time!

---

8 OZ OF LEAN 100% GRASS-FED GROUND BEEF

1 TSP BLACK PEPPER

1 TSP GARLIC POWDER

1 TSP COCONUT OIL

1 ONION, SLICED

2 TBSP BALSAMIC VINEGAR

1 LARGE TOMATO CUT INTO SLICES (OPTIONAL)

1 AVOCADO, SLICED

---

1. Mix the ground beef with the pepper and garlic powder.
2. Heat a skillet on a medium-high heat, and then add the coconut oil.
3. Sauté the onions for 5-10 minutes until browned.
4. Then add in the balsamic vinegar and sauté for another 5 minutes.
5. Turn off the heat and place onions to one side.
6. Form burger shapes with the ground beef using the palms of your hands, add to the skillet and sauté on each side for about 5-6 minutes or until thoroughly cooked through and no longer pink in the middle. Remove from the skillet.
7. Rest on a wired tray while you assemble your burger on your serving plates by adding sliced tomato, avocado and onions on the top.
8. You can serve as a bun-less burger with a side salad or with a 100% wholegrain burger bun.
9. Enjoy.

MAKE YOUR OWN PIZZA

SERVES 4   PREP TIME: 10 MINUTES   COOK TIME: 40 MINUTES

If you thought you had to give up pizza then you can think again!

FOR THE BASE:

1 CUP TAPIOCA STARCH

1/2 CUP COCONUT FLOUR

2 FREE RANGE EGGS

1 CUP WATER

FOR THE TOPPING:

1/4 RED ONION, FINELY DICED

1 CLOVE GARLIC, MINCED

1/2 CAN CHOPPED TOMATOES

1 SPRIG ROSEMARY

1 SPRIG BASIL

2 BEEF TOMATOES, SLICED

1 JALAPEÑO, SLICED

1/2 CUP LEAN MEAT OF YOUR CHOICE, COOKED AND SLICED

1/2 CUP WATERCRESS OR SPINACH

---

1. Heat oven to 375°f/190°c/Gas Mark 5.
2. Get a bowl and mix together all of the ingredients for the base until a smooth dough is formed, adding a little more water if necessary.
3. Roll the dough into a pizza base (don't worry if it's not perfect!)
4. Sauté onions and garlic over a medium heat and add chopped tomatoes and herbs, cooking for 5-10 minutes.
5. Layer the base with the tomato sauce, jalapeño, tomato slices and meat pieces and then bake in the oven for 30 minutes on a slatted rack.
6. Ensure the base is cooked through and not soggy before removing from the oven.
7. Transfer to a chopping board, cut into eighths, and then serve immediately with the watercress or spinach scattered on top.
8. Enjoy.

LOVELY LAMB BURGERS & MINTY YOGURT

SERVES 2   PREP TIME: 5 MINUTES   COOK TIME: 20 MINUTES

A lighter alternative to a classic beef burger which tastes delicious with this minty yogurt dip.

---

8 OZ LEAN GROUND LAMB

1 CLOVE OF GARLIC, MINCED

1 TBSP FRESH ROSEMARY, FINELY CHOPPED

1/2 CUP EXTRA VIRGIN OLIVE OIL

1/2 CUP OF LOW FAT GREEK YOGURT

1 LEMON, JUICED

1/4 CUCUMBER, CHOPPED

1/2 BUNCH FRESH MINT

1/2 CUP ARUGULA

---

1. Mix together the ground lamb, garlic, rosemary and half of the olive oil until combined, and then shape 1 inch thick patties with your hands.
2. (Wet your hands first to prevent sticking).
3. Heat the rest of the oil in a skillet over a medium-high heat, and sear the patties for 1 minute on each side.
4. Cook for 8 minutes on each side until they are thoroughly cooked throughout.
5. Mix the yogurt, lemon juice, cucumber and mint together.
6. Serve a dollop of the yogurt dip on top of each lamb burger with a side salad of arugula.
7. Enjoy.

SLOW COOKED BEEF BRISKET

SERVES 4   PREP TIME: 10 MINUTES   COOK TIME: 4 HOURS SLOW COOKER

Tempting and tender, this is a real treat!

---

1 TBSP MUSTARD

1 SPRIG OF THYME

1 SPRIG OF ROSEMARY

2 CLOVES GARLIC, MINCED

1/4 CUP EXTRA VIRGIN OLIVE OIL

1/4 TSP GROUND PEPPER

16 OZ OF 100 GRASS FED BEEF BRISKET WITH THE FAT TRIMMED

1 ONION, SLICED

1 CUP CARROTS, SLICED

2 CUPS CHOPPED TOMATOES/BROTH

---

1. Heat oven to 300°F/150°C/Gas Mark 2.
2. Use a fork to make a paste by mashing the mustard, thyme and rosemary with the garlic before mixing in the oil and pepper.
3. Pour the mixture over the brisket and rub in well.
4. Place half of the veggies onto the bottom of a baking dish.
5. Place the beef on top of the vegetables.
6. Scatter around the rest of the vegetables and pour over the chopped tomatoes/broth.
7. Cover and bake in the oven or slow cooker for about 3-4 hours, or until very tender.
8. Serve with your favorite side.

SUPER LAMB SHOULDER WITH APRICOT & ZUCCHINIS

SERVES 4   PREP TIME: 10 MINUTES   COOK TIME: 4-5 HOURS

A very quick and easy, healthy lamb recipe to liven up your day!

---

1 LEAN LAMB SHOULDER

4 TBSP. EXTRA VIRGIN OLIVE OIL

5 SPRIGS ROSEMARY

3 SPRIGS THYME

1 TSP BLACK PEPPER

1/2 CUP APRICOTS

HANDFUL OF ARUGULA

2 ZUCCHINIS, CHOPPED

2 GARLIC CLOVES, CHOPPED

HANDFUL OF CHOPPED CILANTRO

---

1. Preheat oven to its highest setting.
2. Prepare the meat by trimming the fat layer off.
3. Rub the lamb with 3 tbsp olive oil, rosemary and thyme as well as a little black pepper.
4. Line a baking tray with the apricots and place lamb shoulder on top.
5. Cover the dish with aluminum foil or a baking lid.
6. Turn the oven down to 325°f/170°c/Gas Mark 3.
7. Cook for 4-5 hours, remove and rest.
8. Now, add 1 tbsp oil to a skillet and heat over a medium heat.
9. Throw in the zucchinis and garlic and sauté for 5-6 minutes until soft.
10. Stir in the cilantro.
11. Serve the lamb on a bed of the veg, drizzling over the juices from the bottom of the pan, and enjoy!

CHILI BEEF & BROCCOLI CURRY

SERVES 4   PREP TIME: 2 MINUTES   COOK TIME: 50 MINUTES

Scrumptious curry, yet so simple to make!

- 2 TBSP OF COCONUT OIL
- 2 GARLIC CLOVES, MINCED
- 16 OZ OF 100% GRASS-FED SIRLOIN OR FILLET STEAK, DICED
- 2 TBSP OF GINGER, GRATED
- 1 TBSP OF BLACK PEPPER

- 1 TBSP OF LEMON JUICE
- 1 CUP OF HOMEMADE CHICKEN BROTH
- 1 CUP CARROTS, CHOPPED
- 1 ONION, CHOPPED
- 1 RED CHILI, FINELY CHOPPED
- 1 CUP OF BROCCOLI

---

1. Heat the coconut oil and garlic in a large pan over a high heat.
2. Add the diced steak to the pan and brown both sides for around 5-6 minutes.
3. Once brown, remove the beef and place to one side.
4. Mix the ginger, pepper, lemon juice and ¼ of the homemade chicken broth to a measuring jug. .
5. Add the beef back into the pan then pour over the broth.
6. Now add the chopped onions and chili to the pan.
7. Bring the liquid to boiling point, then turn down to a simmer for 40 minutes or until piping hot and beef is cooked through.
8. Add the broccoli and chopped carrots into the pan after 20 minutes.
9. Serve right away and enjoy.

MIGHTY HERB PORK MEATBALLS

SERVES 2   PREP TIME: 5 MINUTES   COOK TIME: 30 MINUTES

These meatballs are made with lean pork so are less inflammatory than beef. They also taste magnificent!

---

8 OZ LEAN PORK MINCE

3 TBSP EXTRA VIRGIN OLIVE OIL

1 GARLIC CLOVE, CRUSHED

1/4 CUP 100% WHOLEGRAIN BREAD CRUMBS (GF)

1 TSP DRIED THYME

1 TSP DRIED BASIL

1 CUP 100% WHOLEGRAIN OR GLUTEN FREE SPAGHETTI TO SERVE

FOR THE SAUCE:

1 TBSP EXTRA VIRGIN OLIVE OIL

1 RED ONION, FINELY CHOPPED

1 CUP CANNED CHOPPED TOMATOES

1/2 CUP WATER

1 TBSP FRESH BASIL

---

1. Mix the pork mince, 1 tbsp oil, garlic, breadcrumbs and herbs in a bowl. Season with a little black pepper and separate into 8 balls, rolling with the palms of your hands.
2. Heat 1 tbsp oil in a pan over a medium heat and add onions, sautéing for a few minutes until softened.
3. Add the tomatoes and ½ cup water.
4. Cover and lower heat to a simmer for 15 minutes.
5. Meanwhile, in a separate pan, heat 1 tbsp oil and add the meatballs, turning carefully to brown the surface of each. Continue this for 5-7 minutes before adding to the sauce and simmering for a further 5 minutes.
6. Portion up the meatballs with a helping of sauce.
7. Sprinkle with a little freshly torn basil and enjoy.

HANDY TIP: Try serving with wholegrain (GF) spaghetti or as a tapas dish.

HANDY TIP 2: Alternatively use 1 cup broth and 1/2 cup water for the sauce instead of tomatoes.

THAI BEEF WITH COCONUT MILK

SERVES 2   PREP TIME: 5 MINUTES   COOK TIME: 35 MINUTES

Fast and fresh!

---

2 TBSP COCONUT OIL

1 TSP CRUSHED GARLIC

1 ONION CUT INTO WEDGES

8 OZ ROUND STEAK, CUT INTO STRIPS

2 SLICED CELERY STALKS

2 CUPS BROCCOLI FLORETS

1 RED CAPSICUM, CUT INTO PIECES (OPTIONAL)

1 CUP COCONUT MILK

1 TBSP RED CHILI FLAKES

1/2 CUP BEEF STOCK

BLACK PEPPER TO TASTE

1 LIME

---

1. Heat a wok over a medium heat, and then add the oil, garlic and onion, cooking for 1 minute.
2. Add the beef into the wok and cook for 3 minutes.
3. Add in the celery, broccoli, and capsicum into the wok and stir-fry for 4 minutes.
4. Add the coconut milk, beef stock, chili flakes and black pepper and simmer for 20-25 minutes or until beef is cooked through.
5. Serve hot with your choice of greens and a wedge of lime to squeeze!

LUSH LAMB & ROSEMARY CASSEROLE

SERVES 2   PREP TIME: 5 MINUTES   COOK TIME: 1 HOUR 15 MINUTES

Hearty, wholesome and super easy to make!

---

1 TBSP OF OLIVE OIL	4 CUPS OF HOMEMADE CHICKEN BROTH
2 LEAN LAMB FILLETS, CUBED	1/2 CUP KALE
1 ONION, CHOPPED	1 TSP DRIED ROSEMARY
2 CARROTS, CUBED	2 CANS RINSED AND DRAINED CANNELLINI BEANS
	1 TSP OF CHOPPED PARSLEY

---

1. In a large pot, heat the olive oil over a medium high heat.
2. Add the lamb and cook for 5 minutes until browned.
3. Add the chopped onion and carrots.
4. Leave to cook for another 5 minutes until the vegetables begin to soften.
5. Add the chicken broth, kale and rosemary.
6. Cover the pot and leave to simmer on a low heat for 1-hour until the lamb is tender and fully cooked through.
7. Add the cannellini beans 15 minutes before the end of the cooking time.
8. Plate up and serve with the chopped parsley to garnish.
9. Enjoy.

POULTRY MAIN DISHES

TOMATO & OLIVE CHICKEN FIESTA

SERVES 2   PREP TIME: 5 MINUTES   COOK TIME: 40 MINUTES

A taste of the Mediterranean!

---

2 FREE RANGE SKINLESS CHICKEN BREASTS

1 ONION, ROUGHLY CHOPPED

2 GARLIC CLOVES, CHOPPED

2 CANS CHOPPED TOMATOES

1 TBSP BALSAMIC VINEGAR

8 GREEN OLIVES, CHOPPED

2 CUPS HOMEMADE CHICKEN BROTH

HANDFUL OF FRESH BASIL LEAVES

A PINCH OF BLACK PEPPER

---

1. Preheat oven to 375°F/190 °C/Gas Mark 5.
2. Add all of the ingredients into a deep oven or casserole dish.
3. Place in the oven for 35-40 minutes or until chicken is cooked throughout.
4. Plate up and serve with the remaining basil as a garnish.
5. Enjoy with quinoa or wholegrain bread to mop up the lovely juices.

CAJUN CHICKEN & PRAWN

SERVES 2   PREP TIME: 5 MINUTES   COOK TIME: 35 MINUTES

A very tasty recipe, inspired by Cajun cuisine.

- 1 TSP CAYENNE PEPPER
- 1 TSP CHILI POWDER
- 1 TSP PAPRIKA
- 1/4 TSP CHILI POWDER
- 1 TSP DRIED OREGANO
- 1 TSP DRIED THYME
- 1 TBSP EXTRA VIRGIN OLIVE OIL
- 2 FREE RANGE SKINLESS CHICKEN BREASTS, CHOPPED

- 1 ONION, CHOPPED
- 2 GARLIC CLOVES, CRUSHED
- 10 FRESH OR FROZEN KING PRAWNS
- 1 CUP WHOLEGRAIN RICE
- 1 CAN CHOPPED TOMATOES/1 CUP WATER
- 1 CUP HOMEMADE CHICKEN BROTH
- 1 TSP FRESH CILANTRO, CHOPPED

---

1. Mix the spices and herbs in a bowl to form your Cajun spice mix.
2. Grab a large pan and add the olive oil, heating on a medium heat.
3. Add the chicken and brown each side for around 4-5 minutes. Place to one side.
4. Add the onion to the pan and fry until soft.
5. Add the garlic, prawns and Cajun seasoning to the pan and cook for around 5 minutes or until prawns become opaque.
6. Add the rice along with the chopped tomatoes, chicken and chicken broth to the pan.
7. Cover and allow to simmer for around 25 minutes or until the rice is soft and cooked through.
8. Serve and enjoy with a sprinkle of fresh cilantro.

HANDY TIP: multiply the quantities of the spices to make a Cajun spice mix that you can use again –just keep in a sealable jar or Tupperware somewhere dry!

HEALTHY TURKEY GUMBO

SERVES 4-6   PREP TIME: 5 MINUTES   COOK TIME: 2 HOURS

An all-American staple that you can enjoy the anti-inflammatory way!

---

1 WHOLE TURKEY

1 ONION, QUARTERED

A STALK OF CELERY, CHOPPED

3 CLOVES GARLIC, CHOPPED

1 TBSP EXTRA VIRGIN OLIVE OIL

1/2 CUP OKRA

1 CAN CHOPPED TOMATOES

1-2 BAY LEAVES

BLACK PEPPER TO TASTE

---

1. Take the first four ingredients and add (with water to cover) to a stockpot, over a high heat.
2. Bring to the boil, then lower the heat and simmer for 45-50 minutes or until turkey is cooked through.
3. Remove the turkey and strain the broth - place to one side.
4. While turkey is cooking, grab a skillet and then heat the oil on a medium heat.
5. Add the okra for 5-10 minutes.
6. Add to the turkey broth in the pan and heat over a low heat.
7. Now slice the turkey meat from earlier.
8. Add the tomatoes and half the turkey meat to the broth and stir.
9. Add the bay leaves and continue to cook for an hour or until sauce has thickened.
10. Season with black pepper and enjoy.

HANDY TIP: allow the extra turkey meat to cool before adding to a sealed container and refrigerating for 2-3 days. Tastes great as part of a quinoa salad or in your sandwiches the next day!

CHINESE ORANGE-SPICED DUCK BREASTS

SERVES 2   PREP TIME: 4 MINUTES   COOK TIME: 20 MINUTES

This citrus infused duck is bursting with flavor and easier to cook than you might think!

---

2 DUCK BREASTS, SKIN REMOVED

1 TSP EXTRA VIRGIN OLIVE OIL

1 WHITE ONION, SLICED

3 CLOVES GARLIC, MINCED

2 TSP GINGER, GRATED

1 TSP CINNAMON

1 TSP CLOVES

1 ORANGE – ZEST AND JUICE (RESERVE THE WEDGES)

2 BOK CHOY PLANTS, LEAVES SEPARATED

---

1. Add the duck breasts to a dry hot pan, cooking for 5-7 minutes on each side or until cooked through to your liking.
2. Remove and place to one side.
3. Add olive oil to a clean pan and sauté the onions with the garlic, ginger, cinnamon and cloves for 3-4 minutes.
4. Add the juice and zest of the orange and continue to sauté for 3-5 minutes.
5. Add the duck and bok choy and heat through until wilted and duck is piping hot.
6. Carefully slice the duck breasts and serve on a bed of bok choy, drizzle over any juices left in the pan.
7. Enjoy!

HARISSA SPICED CHICKEN TRAY-BAKE

SERVES 4   PREP TIME: 10 MINUTES   COOK TIME: 35 MINUTES

When time is limited but you don't want flavor to be...this should be a week night staple in any home!

FOR THE HARISSA PASTE:

1 RED PEPPER, DICED

1 TSP DRIED RED CHILLI,
1 GARLIC CLOVE, MINCED

1 TSP CARAWAY SEEDS, CRUSHED
1 TSP GROUND CUMIN

1 TSP FRESH OR DRIED CILANTRO

1 TBSP TOMATO PURÉE (NO ADDED SALT OR SUGAR)

1 TBSP EXTRA VIRGIN OLIVE OIL

1/2 CUP OF LOW-FAT GREEK YOGURT

4 FREE RANGE SKINLESS CHICKEN BREASTS, DICED

1 SMALL BUTTER NUT SQUASH, CHOPPED AND PEELED

2 RED ONIONS, CHOPPED

---

1. Preheat oven to 375°F/190 °C/Gas Mark 5.
2. In a bowl, combine the ingredients for the harissa paste and then add 3 tbsp yogurt.
3. Coat the chicken breasts with the mixture, cover and marinate in the refrigerator if you have time.
4. When ready to cook, scatter the chicken pieces, chopped butternut squash and onions with the remaining harissa paste over a baking tray and place in the oven for 35 minutes or until the chicken is cooked right through.
5. Plate up and serve with the remaining yogurt.
6. Enjoy.

HANDY TIP: double up the harissa spices and save some for cooking later on – it tastes great on fish, chicken, turkey and even simple roast Mediterranean vegetables.

TERRIFIC TURKEY BURGERS

SERVES 2   PREP TIME: 5 MINUTES   COOK TIME: 35 MINUTES

Healthy turkey burgers - great if you've decided to cut out red meat.

---

8 OZ LEAN GROUND TURKEY MEAT

1 WHITE ONIONS, MINCED

1 CARROT, SHREDDED

2 CELERY STALKS, FINELY CHOPPED

1 RED BELL PEPPER, FINELY CHOPPED (OPTIONAL)

1 TBSP DILL

1 TSP CILANTRO

1 TSP DRY MUSTARD

2 TBSP OLIVE OIL

PINCH OF BLACK PEPPER TO TASTE

---

1. Preheat oven to 390°F/200 °C/Gas Mark 6.
2. Mix all the vegetables well in a mixing bowl.
3. Use your hands to shape 2-4 patties depending on how big you like them!
4. Place the patties on a lightly oiled baking tray and bake in the oven for 25-30 minutes or until meat is cooked through (flip half way).
5. Turn up the broiler and broil for the last 5 minutes for a golden and crispy edge.
6. Serve on a bed of your favorite salad and enjoy.

HANDY TIP: an egg helps the burger mixture stick together - try adding if you can eat eggs.

SUPER SESAME CHICKEN NOODLES

SERVES 2   PREP TIME: 10 MINUTES   COOK TIME: 20 MINUTES

Go ahead and mix things up with this tasty recipe.

---

2 TSP COCONUT OIL

2 FREE RANGE SKINLESS CHICKEN BREASTS, CHOPPED

1 CUP RICE/BUCKWHEAT NOODLES SUCH AS JAPANESE UDON

1 CARROT, CHOPPED

1/2 CUP SNOW PEAS

1 TSP SESAME SEEDS

1 THUMB SIZED PIECE OF GINGER, MINCED

1/2 ORANGE, JUICED

---

1. Heat 1 tsp oil in a skillet over a medium heat.
2. Sauté the chopped chicken breast for about 10-15 minutes or until cooked through.
3. Now place the noodles, carrots and peas in a pot of boiling water for about 5 minutes. Drain.
4. In a bowl, mix together the ginger, sesame seeds, 1 tsp oil and orange juice to make your dressing.
5. Combine chicken, noodles and the dressing. Toss to coat.
6. Serve warm or chilled and enjoy.

LEBANESE CHICKEN KEBABS AND HUMMUS

SERVES 4   PREP TIME: 10 MINUTES COOK TIME: 25 MINUTES

Spicy chicken recipe inspired by Lebanese cuisine.

FOR THE CHICKEN:

1 CUP LEMON JUICE

8 GARLIC CLOVES, MINCED

1 TBSP THYME, FINELY CHOPPED

1 TBSP PAPRIKA

2 TSP GROUND CUMIN

1 TSP CAYENNE PEPPER

4 FREE RANGE SKINLESS CHICKEN BREASTS, CUBED

4 METAL KEBAB SKEWERS

LEMON WEDGES TO GARNISH

FOR THE HUMMUS:

1 CAN CHICKPEAS/ 1 CUP DRIED CHICKPEAS SOAKED OVERNIGHT

2 TBSP TAHINI PASTE

1 LEMON, JUICED

1 TSP TURMERIC

1 TSP BLACK PEPPER

2 TBSP OLIVE OIL

1. Whisk the lemon juice, garlic, thyme, paprika, cumin, and cayenne pepper in a bowl.
2. Skewer the chicken cubes using kebab sticks (metal).
3. Baste the chicken on each side with the marinade, cover, and marinate for as long as possible in the fridge (the lemon juice will tenderize the meat).
4. When ready to cook, preheat the oven to 400°F/200 °C/Gas Mark 6.
5. Bake for 20-25 minutes or until chicken is thoroughly cooked through.
6. Prepare the hummus by adding the ingredients to a blender and whizzing up until smooth. If it is a little thick and chunky, add a little water to loosen the mix.
7. Serve the chicken kebabs, garnished with the lemon wedges and the hummus on the side.
8. Enjoy.

ITALIAN CHICKEN & ZUCCHINI SPAGHETTI

SERVES 2   PREP TIME: 10 MINUTES   COOK TIME: 30 MINUTES

Fresh and simple, yet mouthwatering and amazing.

FOR THE CHICKEN:

1 TBSP EXTRA VIRGIN OLIVE OIL

JUICE OF 1/2 LEMON

1 CLOVE GARLIC, CRUSHED

1/2 TSP DRIED OREGANO

PINCH OF BLACK PEPPER

2 FREE RANGE SKINLESS CHICKEN BREAST, SLICED

FOR THE PASTA:

3 ZUCCHINIS

1 TSP EXTRA VIRGIN OLIVE OIL

---

1. Preheat oven to 400°F/200°C/Gas Mark 6.
2. Combine 1 tbsp olive oil, lemon juice, garlic, oregano and pepper and coat the chicken slices.
3. Line a baking sheet with foil or parchment paper.
4. Layer the chicken strips and cook for 25-30 minutes or until cooked through.
5. Meanwhile, prepare your zucchini by slicing into thin spaghetti strips – use a mandolin or spiralyzer and leave in a colander to drain for 10 minutes.
6. When chicken is cooked, remove from the oven and place to one side.
7. Boil a pan of water on a medium heat.
8. Add your zucchini spaghetti to the water and boil for one minute before immediately draining.
9. Plate and serve, layering half the chicken on top and drizzling with 1 tsp olive oil and a little extra black pepper.
10. Enjoy!

GREEK FENNEL & OLIVE BAKED CHICKEN

SERVES 4-6   PREP TIME: 10 MINUTES   COOK TIME: 1 HOUR

A taste of the Aegean sea!

---

1 WHOLE FREE RANGE CHICKEN

1 TSP BLACK PEPPER

2 TBSP EXTRA VIRGIN OLIVE OIL

2 LEMONS

3 CLOVES GARLIC, MINCED

1 TBSP OREGANO, CHOPPED

1 FENNEL BULB, SLICED

2 WHITE SWEET POTATOES, PEELED AND CUBED

1/3 CUP PITTED BLACK OR KALAMATA OLIVES, HALVED

---

1. Preheat oven to 375°F/190 °C/Gas Mark 5.
2. Pat the chicken dry with kitchen towel and place on a lined baking tray.
3. Use a sharp knife to slide underneath the skin and create a pocket. Sprinkle pepper underneath the skin.
4. Mix 1 tbsp olive oil, lemon zest of 1 lemon and juice of 2 lemons with the garlic and oregano (save the lemon wedges).
5. Pour this into the pocket under the skin to marinate for as little or as much time as you have (don't worry if it drizzles out of the pocket).
6. Toss the fennel, sweet potato and olives, 1 tbsp oil and the lemon wedges together in a separate bowl.
7. Scatter the fennel mix around the base of the chicken.
8. Bake for 1 hour or following package guidelines to ensure chicken is thoroughly cooked through.
9. Remove from the oven and allow to rest before carving into servings of the breasts, legs, thighs and any extra flaky meat you can cut away.
10. Serve immediately with a helping of the vegetables and juices from the base of the dish.
11. Enjoy.

ROSEMARY CHICKEN & SWEET POTATO STEW

SERVES 4   PREP TIME: 5 MINUTES   COOK TIME: 40 MINUTES

A tasty and wholesome low fat & low carb chicken recipe.

---

1 TSP EXTRA VIRGIN OLIVE OIL

1 WHITE ONION, CHOPPED

2 GARLIC CLOVES, SLICED

1 CAN OF CHOPPED TOMATOES

2 TBSP CHOPPED ROSEMARY LEAVES

A PINCH OF BLACK PEPPER

4 FREE RANGE SKINLESS CHICKEN THIGHS

4 SWEET POTATOES, PEELED AND CUBED

2 TBSP BASIL LEAVES

---

1. Preheat oven to 375°F/190 °C/Gas Mark 5.
2. Heat oil in a large pan over a medium heat and add the onion and garlic and cook for 5 minutes or until soft.
3. Pour in the chopped tomatoes, rosemary and pepper and cook for around 15 minutes until the mixture starts to thicken.
4. Place the chicken and sweet potato into a baking dish and pour over the sauce before transferring to the oven. Top up with a little water to ensure the chicken and potatoes are covered.
5. Bake for 20-25 minutes or until the chicken is cooked right through.
6. Check every now and then to ensure it doesn't dry up, adding a little water if necessary.
7. Sprinkle the basil over to serve.
8. Enjoy.

HANDY TIP: double up to make in bulk and save the rest in a sealable container for 2-3 days. This also tastes amazing whizzed up in a blender as a soup!

NUTTY PESTO CHICKEN SUPREME

SERVES 2   PREP TIME: 10 MINUTES   COOK TIME: 30 MINUTES

Homemade rustic pesto tastes delicious with poultry, fish and vegetables.

---

2 FREE RANGE SKINLESS CHICKEN OR TURKEY BREASTS

1 CUP CRUSHED MACADAMIAS/ ALMONDS/WALNUTS OR A COMBINATION

1 BUNCH OF FRESH BASIL

1/2 CUP RAW SPINACH

2 TBSP EXTRA VIRGIN OLIVE OIL

1/2 CUP LOW FAT HARD CHEESE (OPTIONAL)

---

1. Preheat oven to 350°f/170°c/Gas Mark 4.
2. Take the chicken breasts and use a meat pounder to 'thin' each breast into a 1cm thick escalope.
3. Reserve a handful of the nuts before adding the rest of the ingredients and a little black pepper to a blender or pestle and mortar and blend until smooth (you can leave this a little chunky for a rustic feel if you wish).
4. Add a little water if the pesto needs loosening.
5. Coat the chicken in the pesto.
6. Bake for at least 30 minutes in the oven, or until chicken is completely cooked through.
7. Top each chicken escalope with the remaining nuts and place under the broiler for 5 minutes for a crispy topping to complete.
8. Serve with your choice of side salad or vegetables and enjoy.

SEAFOOD MAIN DISHES

GINGER & CHILI SEA BASS FILLETS

SERVES 2   PREP TIME: 5 MINUTES   COOK TIME: 10 MINUTES

Fresh and spicy, this sea bass dish is a must-try!

---

1 TBSP EXTRA VIRGIN OLIVE OIL

1 TSP BLACK PEPPER

2 SEA BASS FILLETS

1 RED CHILI, DE-SEEDED AND THINLY SLICED

1 GARLIC CLOVE, THINLY SLICED

1 TSP GINGER, PEELED AND CHOPPED

2 GREEN ONION STEMS, SLICED

---

1. Get a skillet and heat the oil on a medium-high heat.
2. Sprinkle black pepper over the sea bass and score the skin of the fish a few times with a sharp knife.
3. Add the sea bass fillet to the very hot pan with the skin side down.
4. Cook for 5 minutes and turn over.
5. Cook for a further 2 minutes.
6. Remove sea bass from the pan and rest.
7. Add the chili, garlic and ginger and cook for approximately 2 minutes or until golden.
8. Remove from the heat and add the green onions.
9. Scatter the vegetables over your sea bass to serve.
10. Try with a steamed sweet potato or side salad.
11. Enjoy.

SMOKED HADDOCK & PEA RISOTTO

SERVES 2   PREP TIME: 4 MINUTES   COOK TIME: 40 MINUTES

Risotto is amazing but most recipes call for risotto rice - use brown for an anti-inflammatory dish!

1 TBSP EXTRA VIRGIN OLIVE OIL

1 WHITE ONION, FINELY DICED

2 CUPS BROWN RICE

4 CUPS VEGETABLE STOCK
1 CUP FRESH SPINACH LEAVES

1 CUP OF FROZEN PEAS

2 SMOKED HADDOCK FILLETS SKINLESS, BONELESS

3 TBSP LOW FAT GREEK YOGURT (OPTIONAL)

A PINCH OF BLACK PEPPER

4 LEMON WEDGES

1 CUP OF ARUGULA

1. Heat the oil in a large pan on a medium heat.
2. Sauté the chopped onion for 5 minutes until soft before adding in the rice and stirring for 1-2 minutes.
3. Add half of the stock and stir slowly.
4. Slowly add the stock whilst stirring for up to 20-30 minutes (this is a bit of a workout!)
5. Stir in the spinach and peas to the risotto.
6. Place the fish on top of the rice, cover and steam on a medium heat for 10 minutes.
7. Use your fork to break up the fish fillets and stir into the rice with the yogurt.
8. Sprinkle with freshly ground pepper to serve and a squeeze of fresh lemon.
9. Garnish with the lemon wedges and serve with the arugula.
10. Enjoy.

TASTY NUTTY TROUT

SERVES 2   PREP TIME: 5 MINUTES   COOK TIME: 15 MINUTES

This fish is so nutritious and the nuts add a lovely taste and texture!

---

1 TBSP EXTRA VIRGIN OLIVE OIL

1/2 CUP WHOLE WHEAT BREADCRUMBS

1/2 CUP FRESH PARSLEY, FINELY CHOPPED

ZEST AND JUICE OF 1 LEMON

1/2 CUP CHOPPED ALMONDS

2 TROUT FILLETS

---

1. Preheat the broiler to a high heat.
2. Lightly oil a baking tray.
3. Mix the breadcrumbs, parsley, lemon zest and juice and nuts together in a shallow dish.
4. Lay the fillets skin side down onto the oiled baking tray and then flip over so that both sides of your fish are coated in the oil.
5. Now, dip the fillets into the nut mixture on both sides to coat.
6. Return to the baking tray.
7. Broil for 6-7 minutes on each side and serve with a side salad or vegetables of your choice.
8. Enjoy.

PARSLEY & LEMON SPANISH SHRIMP

SERVES 2   PREP TIME: 10 MINUTES   COOK TIME: 20 MINUTES

This shrimp is influenced by Spanish paella dishes and is really easy to prepare!

---

2 CUPS BROWN RICE

4 CUPS OF WATER

1 TBSP EXTRA VIRGIN OLIVE OIL

2 GARLIC CLOVES, CRUSHED

1 WHITE ONION, DICED
1/2 TSP RED PEPPER FLAKES (OPTIONAL)

12 WHOLE SHRIMP, PEELED, DE-VEINED AND THE TAILS STILL INTACT

1 TBSP PARSLEY, CRUSHED

1 LEMON, JUICE AND ZEST

1 LEMON – CUT INTO QUARTERS

---

1. Add the rice and 4 cups of water to a saucepan, bring to a boil over a high heat.
2. Once boiling, lower the heat, cover and simmer for 15 minutes.
3. Meanwhile heat the oil in a skillet on a medium heat and then sauté the garlic, onion and red pepper flakes for 5 minutes until softened and then add the shrimp.
4. Sauté for 5-8 minutes or until shrimp is opaque
5. Drain the rice and return to the heat for a further 2 minutes with the lid on (this will steam the rice and make it lovely and fluffy).
6. Add the rice to the shrimps.
7. Add in the parsley, zest and juice of 1 lemon and mix well.
8. Serve in a wide paella dish if possible or a large serving dish – scatter the lemon wedges around the edge and sprinkle with a little more fresh parsley.
9. Season with black pepper to taste and enjoy.

NUT-CRUST TILAPIA WITH KALE

SERVES 2   PREP TIME: 5 MINUTES   COOK TIME: 15 MINUTES

A perfect blend of crunchy coated fish with iron-rich kale.

---

2 TSP EXTRA VIRGIN OLIVE OIL

2 TBSP LOW FAT HARD CHEESE, GRATED

1/2 CUP ROASTED AND GROUND BRA-ZIL NUTS/HAZELNUTS/ANY OTHER HARD NUT

1/2 CUP 100% WHOLEGRAIN (GF) BREADCRUMBS

2 TSP WHOLE GRAIN MUSTARD

2 TILAPIA FILLETS, SKINLESS

1 CLOVE OF GARLIC, MASHED

1 HEAD OF KALE, CHOPPED

1 TBSP SESAME SEEDS, LIGHTLY TOASTED

---

1. Preheat oven to 350°f/170°c/Gas Mark 4.
2. Lightly oil a baking sheet with 1 tsp extra virgin olive oil.
3. Mix the cheese, breadcrumbs and nuts in a shallow bowl.
4. Spread a thin layer of the mustard over the fish and then dip into the breadcrumb mixture.
5. Transfer to the baking dish.
6. Bake for 12 minutes or until cooked through.
7. Meanwhile, heat 1 tsp oil in a skillet on a medium heat and sauté the garlic for 30 seconds, adding in the kale for a further 5 minutes.
8. Mix in the sesame seeds.
9. Serve the fish at once with the kale on the side and enjoy.

WASABI SALMON BURGERS

SERVES 4   PREP TIME: 5 MINUTES   COOK TIME: 20 MINUTES

Fish burgers a little Japanese kick!

2 CANS OF WILD SALMON, DRAINED

1 BEATEN FREE RANGE EGG

1 TBSP FRESH GINGER, MINCED

2 SCALLIONS, CHOPPED

2 TBSP COCONUT OIL

2 TBSP REDUCED-SALT SOY SAUCE

1 TSP WASABI POWDER

1/2 TSP HONEY

1. Combine the salmon, egg, ginger, scallions and 1 tbsp oil in a bowl and mix well.
2. Use slightly wet hands to form 4 patties.
3. In a separate bowl, add the soy sauce and wasabi powder with the honey and whisk until blended.
4. Heat 1 tbsp oil over a medium heat in a skillet and cook the patties for 4 minutes each side until firm and browned.
5. Glaze the top of each patty with the wasabi mixture and cook for another 15 seconds before you serve.
6. Serve with your favorite side salad or vegetables and enjoy.

SALMON & LIME WITH ARUGULA

SERVES 2   PREP TIME: 5 MINUTES   COOK TIME: 10 MINUTES

Rich in omega-3 and iron, this is super brain food!

FOR THE FISH:

2 SKINLESS SALMON FILLETS

1 TBSP EXTRA VIRGIN OLIVE OIL

1/2 FRESH LIME, JUICED

A PINCH OF BLACK PEPPER TO TASTE

FOR THE SALAD:

4 CUPS BABY ARUGULA LEAVES

1/2 CUP SLIVERED RED ONION

1 CUP CHERRY TOMATOES, CUT INTO HALVES (OPTIONAL)

1 TBSP OLIVE OIL

1 TBSP BALSAMIC VINEGAR

---

1. In a bowl, coat the salmon with the olive oil, lime juice and pepper (if you can, leave for at least 15 minutes up to an hour but don't worry if not).
2. Heat a skillet over a medium heat and cook the salmon, skin-side down, for 4-5 minutes each side or until completely cooked through.
3. Add the arugula, onion and tomatoes with oil and vinegar to a separate bowl and toss.
4. Serve the fish on the bed of salad and enjoy.

SPICY COD BROTH

SERVES 2   PREP TIME: 10 MINUTES   COOK TIME: 20 MINUTES

An aromatic and spicy bowl of goodness.

---

2 BLACK COD FILLETS

A PINCH OF BLACK PEPPER

1 TSP REDUCED SODIUM SOY SAUCE

2 CUPS HOMEMADE CHICKEN/VEG BROTH

1 TSP COCONUT OIL

1 TSP FIVE-SPICE POWDER

1 TBSP OLIVE OIL

3 HEADS OF BOK CHOY

1 CARROT, SLICED

1 TBSP GINGER, MINCED

2 CUPS OF UDON NOODLES

1 GREEN ONION, THINLY SLICED

2 TSP CILANTRO, FINELY CHOPPED

1 TSP SESAME SEEDS

---

1. Rub the fish with pepper.
2. In a bowl, combine soy sauce, 1 cup broth, coconut oil and spice blend. Mix together and place to one side.
3. In a large saucepan, heat the olive oil over a medium heat and add the bok choy, carrot and ginger for 2-3 minutes until the bok choy is dark green and slightly wilted.
4. Add the rest of the reserved broth and heat through.
5. Add the udon noodles and stir, bringing to a simmer.
6. Add the green onion and the fish and cook for 10-15 minutes until fish is tender.
7. Add the fish, noodles and vegetables into serving bowls and pour the broth over the top.
8. Garnish with the cilantro and sesame seeds and serve with chopsticks for real authenticity and enjoy!

HANDY TIP: This works with most types of white fish or even salmon so switch things up according to what's sustainable at the time of cooking!

BAKED GARLIC & LEMON HALIBUT

SERVES 2   PREP TIME: 5 MINUTES   COOK TIME: 15 MINUTES

Garlic is renowned for its anti-inflammatory properties and tastes delicious with this meaty fish.

---

2 HALIBUT FILLETS

A PINCH OF BLACK PEPPER

2 GARLIC CLOVES, PRESSED

2 TBSP OLIVE OIL

4 LEMON WEDGES TO GARNISH

---

1. Preheat oven to 400°f/190°c/Gas Mark 5.
2. Season the fish with the pepper and add to a parchment paper-lined baking dish.
3. Scatter the garlic cloves (no need to peel) around the fish and drizzle with the oil.
4. Squeeze the lemon juice over the fish and scatter the lemon wedges onto the dish.
5. Bake for approximately 15 minutes until the fish is firm and well cooked.
6. Serve and pour over the juices for a delicious garlic feast.
7. Enjoy.

FRESH TUNA STEAK & FENNEL SALAD

SERVES 2   PREP TIME: 5 MINUTES   COOK TIME: 25 MINUTES

The aniseed taste of the fennel blends so well with the delicate peas and the meaty taste of the tuna.

---

2 TUNA STEAKS, EACH 1 INCH THICK

2 TBSP OLIVE OIL

1 TSP CRUSHED BLACK PEPPERCORNS

1 TSP CRUSHED FENNEL SEEDS

1 FENNEL BULB, TRIMMED AND SLICED

1 GARLIC CLOVE, CRUSHED

1/2 CUP WATER

1 LEMON, JUICED

1 TSP FRESH PARSLEY, CHOPPED

---

1. Coat the fish with 1 tbsp oil and then season with peppercorns and fennel seeds. Place to one side.
2. Heat the oil over a medium heat and sauté the fennel bulb slices for 5 minutes or until light brown, stir in the garlic and cook for another minute.
3. Add the water to the pan and cook for 10 minutes until fennel is tender.
4. Stir in the lemon juice and lower heat to a simmer.
5. Meanwhile, heat another skillet and sauté the tuna steaks for about 2-3 minutes each side for medium-rare.
6. (Add 1 minute each side for medium and 2 minutes each side for medium well).
7. Serve the fennel mix with the tuna steaks on top and garnish with the fresh parsley.
8. Enjoy.

SESAME MAHI MAHI & FRUIT SALSA

SERVES 2   PREP TIME: 5 MINUTES   COOK TIME: 20 MINUTES

This fun tropical dish combines a great-tasting fish with a tangy salsa.

FOR THE SALSA:

1 CUP FRESH PINEAPPLE, PEELED AND CUBED

1/2 RED CHILI, FINELY CHOPPED

1 LIME, JUICED

2 TSP CILANTRO, CHOPPED

1 ONION, FINELY CHOPPED

FOR THE FISH:

2 TSP COCONUT OIL

2 MAHI MAHI FILLETS

2 TBSP SESAME SEEDS

---

1. Get a bowl and mix all of the ingredients for the salsa.
2. Drizzle 1 tsp coconut oil on the fillets and coat each side with the sesame seeds.
3. Heat 1 tsp oil over a medium heat and then sauté the fillets for about 8 minutes each side or until the fish is cooked through.
4. Serve with the salsa on the side and enjoy.

SMOKED SALMON HASH BROWNS

SERVES 2   PREP TIME: 5 MINUTES   COOK TIME: 35 MINUTES

A yummy filling and healthy fish dish.

---

3 TBSP EXTRA VIRGIN OLIVE OIL

1 LEEK, CHOPPED

1 LARGE SWEET POTATO, PEELED AND CUBED

4 TSP DILL, CHOPPED

1 TBSP GRATED ORANGE PEEL

1 PACK SMOKED SALMON, SLICED

1'/3 CUP LOW FAT GREEK YOGURT (OPTIONAL)

---

1. Preheat oven to 325°f/150°c/Gas Mark 3.
2. Lightly grease 2 ramekins or circular baking dishes with a little olive oil.
3. Heat the rest of the oil in a skillet over medium heat, and sauté the leeks and the potatoes for 5 minutes.
4. Lower the heat and cook for another 10 minutes until tender.
5. Transfer the potatoes and leeks to a separate bowl and crush with a fork to form a mash (alternatively use a potato masher).
6. Add the dill, orange peel and the salmon and mix well.
7. Fill the ramekins with half the mixture each, patting to compact.
8. Bake for 15 minutes and remove.
9. Serve hash in the ramekin, season and top with a dollop of Greek yogurt (optional).
10. Enjoy.

SCALLOPS WITH CILANTRO & LIME

SERVES 2   PREP TIME: 5 MINUTES   COOK TIME: 5 MINUTES

A luxurious dish.

---

1 TBSP EXTRA SESAME OIL

8 QUEEN OR KING SCALLOPS (ROW ON)

2 LARGE GARLIC CLOVES, FINELY CHOPPED

1 RED CHILI, FINELY CHOPPED

1/2 LIME JUICE

2 TBSP OF CHOPPED CILANTRO

A PINCH OF BLACK PEPPER

---

1. Heat oil in a skillet on a medium to high heat and add scallops for about 1 minute each side until lightly golden.
2. Add the garlic and chili to the skillet and squeeze the lime juice over the scallops.
3. Saute for 2-3 minutes.
4. Remove the scallops and sprinkle the cilantro and black pepper over the top to serve.
5. Enjoy.

GLUTEN-FREE COCONUT SHRIMP BITES

SERVES 2   PREP TIME: 10 MINUTES   COOK TIME:15 MINUTES

A healthy lightly battered shrimp dish.

1/4 CUP COCONUT FLOUR

1/2 TSP CAYENNE PEPPER

1 TSP GARLIC POWDER

2 BEATEN FREE RANGE EGGS

1/2 CUP SHREDDED COCONUT

1/4 CUP ALMOND FLOUR

A PINCH OF BLACK PEPPER TO TASTE

2 CUPS SHRIMP, PEELED AND DE-VEINED

1 CUP ARUGULA OR WATERCRESS

---

1. Preheat oven to 400°f/200°c/Gas Mark 6.
2. Line a baking sheet with parchment paper.
3. Mix the coconut flour, cayenne pepper, and garlic powder in a bowl.
4. In a separate bowl, whisk the eggs.
5. In a third bowl, add the shredded coconut, almond flour and pepper.
6. Dip the shrimp into each dish in consecutive order, and then placc on the baking sheet and bake for 10-15 minutes or until cooked through.
7. Serve piping hot and straight from the oven with a side salad of arugula or water-cress.

SPICY SHARK STEAKS

SERVES 2   PREP TIME: 35 MINUTES   COOK TIME: 40 MINUTES

A taste of the exotic! You can use tuna or monk fish in place of shark.

---

2 TBSP ONION POWDER

2 TSP CHILI POWDER

1 GARLIC CLOVE, MINCED

1/4 CUP WORCESTERSHIRE SAUCE

1 TBSP GROUND BLACK PEPPER

2 TBSP THYME, CHOPPED

2 SHARK STEAKS, SKINLESS

---

1. In a bowl, mix all of the seasoning and spices to form a paste before setting aside.
2. Spread a thin layer of paste on both sides of the fish, cover and chill for 30 minutes (If possible).
3. Preheat oven to 325°f/150°c/Gas Mark 3.
4. Bake the fish in parchment paper for 30-40 minutes, until well cooked.
5. Serve on a bed of quinoa or wholegrain couscous and your favorite salad and enjoy.

CITRUS & HERB SARDINES

SERVES 2 / PREP TIME: 5 MINUTES / COOK TIME: 15 MINUTES

Sardines are a great source of protein as well as omega 3's – they're recommended to eat between 2-6 times a week on the anti-inflammatory diet.

ZEST OF 2 WHOLE LEMONS

HANDFUL OF FLAT-LEAF PARSLEY, CHOPPED

2 GARLIC CLOVES, FINELY CHOPPED

1 TBSP OLIVE OIL

10 SARDINES, SCALED AND CLEANED (8 IF LARGE)

1 CUP OF CANNED CHOPPED TOMATOES (OPTIONAL)

1/2 CAN CHICKPEAS OR BUTTER BEANS, DRAINED AND RINSED

8 CHERRY TOMATOES, HALVED (OPTIONAL)

A PINCH OF BLACK PEPPER

---

1. In a bowl add the lemon zest to the chopped parsley (save a pinch for garnishing) and half of the chopped garlic, ready for later.
2. Put a very large skillet on the hob and heat on high.
3. Now add the oil and once very hot, lay the sardines flat on the pan.
4. Sauté for 3 minutes until golden underneath and turn over to fry for another 3 minutes. Place onto a plate to rest.
5. Sauté the remaining garlic (add another splash of oil if you need to) for 1 min until softened. Pour in the tin of chopped tomatoes, mix and let simmer for 4-5 minutes.
6. If you're avoiding tomatoes just avoid this step and go straight to chickpeas.
7. Tip in the chickpeas or butter beans and fresh tomatoes and stir until heated through.
8. Here's when you add the sardines into the lemon and parsley dressing prepared earlier and add to the pan, cooking for a further 3-4 minutes.
9. Once heated through, serve with a pinch of parsley and remaining lemon zest to garnish.
10. Enjoy.

VEGETARIAN MAIN DISHES

LIME & SATAY TOFU WITH SNOW PEAS

SERVES 2   PREP TIME: 5 MINUTES   COOK TIME: 15 MINUTES

This nutty lime dish is amazing.

---

1 TBSP COCONUT OIL

1 PACK OF DRAINED, PRESSED AND CUBED TOFU

FOR THE SAUCE:

3 TBSP ALMOND MILK

1 TBSP WHOLE ALMOND BUTTER

2 TBSP REDUCED SODIUM OYSTER SAUCE

1 TBSP GARLIC POWDER

1 TSP CHILI FLAKES

1 TSP TOMATO PUREE (NO ADDED SUGAR OR SALT)

1 TSP LIME JUICE

A PINCH OF BLACK PEPPER TO TASTE

1 CUP OF SNOW PEAS

1 CUP UDON NOODLES/BROWN RICE, COOKED

---

1. Heat the oil over a high heat and then sauté the tofu until brown on each side.
2. Place onto paper towels to soak excess moisture and place to one side.
3. Heat the milk in a pan over a medium heat until starting to bubble and then add the almond butter and the rest of the ingredients for the sauce, stirring continuously for 5 minutes until smooth and hot.
4. Add the tofu to the sauce, cooking for 4-5 minutes until heated through.
5. Meanwhile, steam or boil your sugar snap peas for 3-4 minutes.
6. Serve all ingredients piping hot with your choice of cooked udon noodles or brown rice.
7. Enjoy.

LATINO BLACK BEAN STEW

SERVES 4   PREP TIME: 5 MINUTES   COOK TIME: 20 MINUTES

If you're craving the distinct taste of an authentic Mexican meal, this recipe is without the usual grease that comes hand in hand with the takeaway version!

---

1 CUP OF FRESHLY BROWN RICE

1 CUP OF FRESHLY QUINOA

1/2 CUP BLACK BEANS

1/2 CUP OF BLACK OLIVES, HALVED

1 BEEF TOMATO, FINELY CHOPPED (OPTIONAL)

1/2 RED ONION, FINELY CHOPPED

1 LIME, JUICED

1 AVOCADO, SLICED

2 TBSP OF PLAIN NON-FAT GREEK YOGURT

1 LIME, CUT INTO WEDGES

1 TBSP FRESH CILANTRO, FINELY CHOPPED

---

1. Heat a pan of water (2 cups) on a high heat and add brown rice for 15 minutes.
2. Meanwhile, heat a separate pan of water (2 cups) on a high heat and add quinoa, allowing to cook for 15 minutes.
3. Add the black beans to the pan of rice to cook along with the rice.
4. Check most of the water in each pan has been absorbed, drain and cover on the heat for 2 minutes. Turn off heat.
5. Grab a large serving bowl and mix rice, quinoa, beans, olives, tomatoes, red onion and lime juice together.
6. In a separate bowl, crush the avocado into the yogurt with a fork and squeeze any remaining lime juice into the dip.
7. Enjoy your authentic Mexican meal, topped with cilantro, the avocado dip, and the lime wedges to serve.
8. Enjoy.

ZUCCHINI & PEPPER LASAGNA

SERVES 1   PREP TIME: 10 MINUTES   COOK TIME: 1 HOUR

Very low in fat and vegan, this is quick and easy to prepare, using only a few ingredients; it's delicious and very filling too!

1/2 PACK OF SOFT TOFU

1/2 PACK OF FIRM TOFU

1/4 TSP OF GARLIC POWDER

1 CUP OF ALMOND MILK

1 1/2 TBSP OF FRESH BASIL, CHOPPED

JUICE OF 1/2 A LEMON

1 RED PEPPER, DICED (OPTIONAL)

1 CUP BABY SPINACH

1 ZUCCHINI , DICED

1 CAN OF CHOPPED TOMATOES

3 WHOLEGRAIN LASAGNA SHEETS (GF)

A PINCH OF BLACK PEPPER TO TASTE

---

1. Preheat oven to 325°F/170 °C/Gas Mark 3.
2. In a blender, process the soft and firm tofu, garlic powder, almond milk, basil, lemon juice and pepper until smooth.
3. Toss in the spinach and zucchini for the last 30 seconds.
4. Put about 1/3 of the chopped tomatoes at the bottom of an oven dish.
5. Top the sauce with 1 of the lasagna sheets and then 1/3 of the tofu mixture.
6. Repeat the layers finishing with the chopped tomatoes on top.
7. Cook for around 1 hour or until the pasta sheets are soft.
8. Serve with a lovely side salad and enjoy.

TOASTED CUMIN CRUNCH

SERVES 1   PREP TIME: 5 MINUTES   COOK TIME: 10 MINUTES

Cumin seeds are renowned for their anti-inflammatory properties and taste amazing with salads and vegetables.

---

1 TBSP EXTRA VIRGIN OLIVE OIL

1 TSP CRACKED BLACK PEPPERCORNS

1/2 TSP CUMIN SEEDS (WHOLE)

1/2 JALAPEÑO, FINELY CHOPPED

2 CUPS OF GREEN CABBAGE, SLICED

2 CUPS OF CARROTS, GRATED

1 TBSP GROUND CUMIN SEEDS (USE A PESTLE AND MORTAR OR BLENDER)

1 TBSP LIME JUICE

1 TSP CILANTRO, FINELY CHOPPED

---

1. Get a large saucepan, and heat the oil over a medium heat.
2. Cook the peppercorns and the whole cumin seeds for about a minute until browned.
3. Add in the jalapeño and then cook for another 45 seconds until tender.
4. Add in then the cabbage and carrots, cooking for about 5 minutes or until the cabbage starts to soften.
5. Add in the ground cumin seeds and cook for 30 seconds before taking off the heat and stirring in the lime juice and the cilantro.
6. Serve warm and enjoy.

SPICY VEGETABLE BURGERS

SERVES 2   PREP TIME: 2 MINUTES   COOK TIME: 15 MINUTES

Spicy and succulent.

EXTRA FIRM TEMPEH
(1 PACK)

2 TBSP COCONUT OIL

1 TSP OF RED CHILI FLAKES

1/2 RED ONION, DICED

1 RED PEPPER, DICED (OPTIONAL)

1/2 CUP BABY SPINACH

2 100% WHOLEGRAIN BUS (GF)
1/2 CUP ARUGULA

---

1. Heat the broiler to a medium-high heat.
2. Marinate the tempeh in 1 tbsp coconut oil and red chili flakes.
3. Heat 1 tbsp coconut oil in a skillet over a medium heat.
4. Sauté the onion in the skillet for 6-7 minutes or until caramelized.
5. Stir in the pepper and baby spinach for a further 3-4 minutes.
6. Broil the tempeh for around 4 minutes on each side.
7. Lay down the tempeh in the buns and then add the caramelized onion, spinach and diced peppers.
8. Serve immediately while hot with a side of arugula.
9. Enjoy.

SUN DRIED TOMATO & NUT PASTA

SERVES 2   PREP TIME: 5 MINUTES   COOK TIME: 20 MINUTES

A delicious pasta dish.

---

1 CUP 100% WHOLEGRAIN PASTA (GF)

1 CLOVE OF GARLIC, MINCED

1/4 CUP OF WALNUTS, COARSELY CHOPPED

1/2 CUP SUN-DRIED TOMATOES, DRAINED & CHOPPED (OPTIONAL)

1 BUNCH FRESH BASIL, CHOPPED

100G OF LOW-FAT MOZZARELLA CHEESE

2 TBSP OF EXTRA VIRGIN OLIVE OIL

PINCH OF BLACK PEPPER

---

1. Boil a large saucepan of water (2 cups) on a high heat.
2. Add the pasta and cook following directions on the package.
3. While the pasta is cooking, prepare the sauce:
4. Put minced garlic in a bowl.
5. Add walnuts, sun-dried tomatoes, basil, mozzarella and oil.
6. Once the pasta is cooked, drain and add to the sauce.
7. Toss through until the pasta is well coated.
8. Transfer onto a serving plate and sprinkle with a little black pepper.

HANDY TIP: If you're avoiding wheat completely, prepare this dish with spiralyzed zucchini or carrots. Just cook in boiling water for 1-2 minutes and serve as you would pasta!

SPAGHETTI SQUASH & MARINATED TEMPEH

SERVES 2   PREP TIME: 15 MINUTES   COOK TIME: 50 MINUTES

Yummy!

---

3 TBSP OF TAMARI OR REDUCED SODIUM SOY SAUCE

1 PACK OF TEMPEH, DRAINED AND CUBED

2 CLOVES OF GARLIC, CHOPPED FINELY

1 SPAGHETTI SQUASH OR PUMPKIN, HALVED AND DE-SEEDED

1 CAN OF CHOPPED TOMATOES

1 CUP SMALL BROCCOLI FLORETS

1/2 CUP OF BABY SPINACH

---

1. Preheat the oven to 375°F/190 °C/Gas Mark 5.
2. Get a medium-sized bowl and toss together the tamari, tempeh, garlic.
3. Marinate for as long as you can and up to overnight if possible.
4. When ready to cook, grab a large baking dish and arrange the squash halves with the cut side down and pour half a cup of water into the dish.
5. Bake for around 45 minutes or until tender and remove the dish from the oven.
6. Turn the squash over and allow to slightly cool.
7. Get a large skillet and heat oil over a medium heat.
8. Add tempeh and cook for 7 to 8 minutes until golden brown, occasionally stirring.
9. Remove the tempeh and keep warm on a plate.
10. Into the skillet, heat chopped tomatoes at medium heat, and then add the broccoli and allow to cook until tender (around 5 minutes.)
11. Stir the spinach in and remove from heat.
12. Use a fork to scrape off spaghetti squash strands onto a platter. Spoon broccoli and hot chopped tomatoes over the dish.
13. Top with the tempeh to serve.
14. Enjoy.

RUSTIC GARLIC & CHIVE QUINOA

SERVES 2   PREP TIME: 5 MINUTES   COOK TIME: 30 MINUTES

A light and simple dish which can be experimented with by adding different flavors and vegetables.

---

1 TBSP EXTRA VIRGIN OLIVE OIL

1/2 WHITE ONION, DICED

4 CLOVES OF GARLIC, MINCED

1/2 CUP OF UNCOOKED QUINOA

1/2 CUP OF KIDNEY BEANS

2 CUPS OF VEGETABLE BROTH

3 GREEN ONION STEMS, DICED

1/4 TSP OF BLACK PEPPER

---

1. In a large pan, sauté the garlic and onion in olive oil over a medium heat until the onions soften.
2. Lower the heat and add the quinoa, kidney beans and vegetable broth.
3. Cover the pan and simmer for around 15 to 20 minutes or until quinoa is soft and liquid is absorbed.
4. Serve with the diced green onion scattered over the quinoa and a little black pepper to taste.
5. Enjoy.

PORTABELLA MUSHROOM CUPS

SERVES 4   PREP TIME: 5 MINUTES   COOK TIME: 10 MINUTES

A high fiber tasty entrée

---

4 LARGE PORTABELLA MUSHROOMS

1/2 CUP OF COOKED QUINOA

1 RED BELL PEPPER, CHOPPED
(OPTIONAL)

1/2 CUCUMBER, CHOPPED

1 GREEN ONION, SLICED

1 TBSP OF DIJON MUSTARD

1 TBSP OF WHITE WINE VINEGAR

1 TBSP OF EXTRA VIRGIN OLIVE OIL

PINCH OF BLACK PEPPER

---

1. Preheat the broiler to a medium-high heat.
2. Combine the cooked quinoa, bell pepper, cucumber, green onion, mustard and white wine vinegar in a separate bowl.
3. Place the portabella mushrooms on a baking sheet and lightly brush with olive oil.
4. Stack the mushroom caps with the quinoa mixture.
5. Place under the broiler for 10 minutes, then serve immediately with black pepper to taste.
6. Enjoy.

INDIAN BROCCOLI RABE & CAULIFLOWER

SERVES 4   PREP TIME: 5 MINUTES   COOK TIME: 25 MINUTES

Lightly spiced vegetables.

---

1 TBSP COCONUT OIL

1 TSP BLACK MUSTARD SEEDS

1 TSP CUMIN SEEDS

1/2 TSP TURMERIC

1 TSP CUMIN POWDER

1/2 TSP CORIANDER POWDER

A PINCH OF BLACK PEPPER TO TASTE
1 ONION, DICED

1 THUMB SIZED PIECE OF GINGER, MINCED

4 GARLIC CLOVES, MINCED

1/2 TSP OF RED CHILI FLAKES

12 BUNCH BROCCOLI RABE (RAPINI)

1/2 CAULIFLOWER, FLORETS

1 TBSP FRESH CILANTRO, CHOPPED TO GARNISH

---

1. In a skillet, add the oil and heat over a medium heat.
2. Add the black mustard seeds, cumin seeds, and the spices (down to black pepper) and stir for 4-5 minutes.
3. Add the onions and stir for a further 5 minutes or until softened.
4. Add the ginger, garlic and red chili flakes, stirring for a further 5 minutes.
5. Now add the broccoli rabe and cauliflower to the mix.
6. Stir until the veg is covered in the spices and then reduce the heat and sauté for about 5-6 minutes.
7. Garnish with cilantro and add pepper to taste and serve.
8. Enjoy.

BOK CHOY & SESAME SEED STIR FRY

SERVES 2   PREP TIME: 2 MINUTES   COOK TIME: 6 MINUTES

A deliciously simple stir fry.

---

1 TBSP COCONUT OIL

2 CLOVES GARLIC, MINCED

1 THUMB SIZED PIECE FRESH GINGER, MINCED

4 BOK CHOY PLANTS, LEAVES SEPARATED

1 TBSP SESAME SEEDS

---

1. Heat the oil in a skillet over a high heat and add in the garlic and ginger.
2. Cook for 1 minute.
3. Add the bok choy and cook for about 5 minutes or until the bok choy stalks are crispy.
4. Season with pepper as needed and sprinkle sesame seeds over to serve.
5. Enjoy.

SALADS

ROASTED BEETS, GOATS CHEESE & EGG SALAD

SERVES 2   PREP TIME: 5 MINUTES   COOK TIME: 25 MINUTES

Beets are a super food that contain nutrients you rarely find in your five portions a day and goats cheese is naturally anti-inflammatory.

1/2 CUP COOKED CHOPPED BEETS (NOT IN VINEGAR)

1 TBSP EXTRA VIRGIN OLIVE OIL + EXTRA FOR BRUSHING

JUICE FROM 1 ORANGE

1 FREE RANGE EGG

2 TBSP LOW FAT GREEK YOGURT

1 TSP DIJON MUSTARD

A FEW STALKS OF DILL, FINELY CHOPPED (FRESH OR DRIED)

1/2 CUP OF BABY GEM LETTUCE

HANDFUL OF WALNUTS

1/4 CUP CRUMBLED GOATS CHEESE

A PINCH BLACK PEPPER

---

1. Preheat oven to 200°C/400°F/Gas Mark 6.
2. Place the beets onto a lightly oiled baking tray with the juice from the orange and sprinkle with pepper.
3. Roast for 20-25 minutes, turning once whilst baking. If it starts to dry out, add a little more olive oil.
4. Meanwhile, boil a pan of water and add the whole egg.
5. Turn down the heat and simmer for 8 minutes (4 minutes if you like your yolks runny) then run under cold water to cool. Peel and halve.
6. Mix the remaining oil, yogurt, mustard and chopped dill together - this is the dressing for your lettuce.
7. Serve the salad with the beetroot,goats cheese and walnuts crumbled over the top.

BULGUR WHEAT, GOATS CHEESE & TABBOULEH SALAD

SERVES 2   PREP TIME: 35 MINUTES   COOK TIME: NA

A variation of the traditional tabbouleh salad, this version features goats' cheese for a tasty twist.

1/2 CUP OF BULGUR WHEAT, UNCOOKED

1 CUP OF WATER, BOILING

1 CAN OF CHICKPEAS, DRAINED

1/4 CUP GOATS' CHEESE, CRUMBLED

8 CHERRY TOMATOES, HALVED (OPTIONAL)

1 LEMON, JUICED

2 TBSP OF FRESH PARSLEY, FINELY

CHOPPED

1/4 TSP OF BLACK PEPPER

1 RED ONION, SLICED THINLY

1/4 CUP TABBOULEH, SPIRALYZED

1. Mix bulgur wheat with 1 cup of boiling water in a large bowl.
2. Cover and set aside for half an hour before draining.
3. Combine the rest of the ingredients in a large bowl.
4. Gently toss to mix well.
5. Serve and enjoy.

SPINACH, ORANGE & CRANBERRY SALAD

SERVES 1   PREP TIME: 5 MINUTES   COOK TIME: NA

Fruity and fun!

---

2 TBSP RED WINE VINEGAR

1 TSP OLIVE OIL

1 CUP FRESH CRANBERRIES, CHOPPED

2 TSP GINGER, PEELED AND GRATED

1 CUP FRESH SPINACH WITH THE LEAVES TRIMMED AND COARSELY CHOPPED

1 ORANGE, PEELED AND SLICED

A PINCH OF BLACK PEPPER TO TASTE

---

1. Grab a salad bowl and mix the vinegar and olive oil until blended and then add in the cranberries and ginger, adding pepper to taste.
2. Add the spinach and orange slices to the dressing and then toss to coat.
3. Chill before serving and enjoy.

KIPPER & CELERY SALAD

SERVES 2   PREP TIME: 2 MINUTES   COOK TIME: NA

Oily fish are recommended up to 6 times per week on an anti-inflammatory diet and taste delicious with celery.

1 CELERY STALK, CHOPPED	1 CLOVE GARLIC, MINCED
1 TBSP FRESH PARSLEY, CHOPPED	1 ONION, MINCED
1/2 CUP LOW FAT GREEK YOGURT	1 CAN OF COOKED KIPPERS
1 LEMON, JUICED	

1. Combine all of the ingredients apart from the kippers into a salad bowl.
2. Drain the kippers and then toss in the dressing mix.
3. Chill before serving or serve right away if you're in a rush.

HANDY TIP: If you have mackerel or sardines, this works just as well.

ON-THE-GO TACO SALAD

SERVES 2   PREP TIME: 5 MINUTES   COOK TIME: 30 MINUTES

This salad can be enjoyed on the side or as a ready to eat lunch on the go!

---

1 TBSP EXTRA VIRGIN OLIVE OIL

2 SKINLESS CHICKEN BREASTS, CHOPPED

2 CARROTS, SLICED

1/2 LARGE ONION, CHOPPED

2 TSP CUMIN SEEDS

1/2 AVOCADO, CHOPPED

1 JUICED LIME

1/2 CUCUMBER, CHOPPED

1/2 CUP FRESH SPINACH, WASHED

2 MASON JARS

---

1. In a skillet, heat up the oil on a medium heat and then cook the chicken for 10-15 minutes until browned and cooked through.
2. Remove and place to one side to cool.
3. Add the carrots and onion and continue to cook for 5-10 minutes or until soft.
4. Add the cumin seeds to a separate pan over a high heat and toast until they're brown before crushing them in a pestle and mortar or blender.
5. Put them into the pan with the veggies and turn off the heat.
6. Add the avocado and lime juice into a food processor and blend until creamy.
7. Layer the jar with half of the avocado and lime mixture, then the cumin roasted veggies, and then the chicken.
8. Top with the cucumber spinach and serve immediately or save in the fridge for later.

SIZZLING SALMON & GREEN SALAD

SERVES 2   PREP TIME: 2 MINUTES   COOK TIME: 10 MINUTES

A summer time staple.

---

2 SKINLESS SALMON FILLETS	2 CUPS OF SEASONAL GREENS
1 LEMON, JUICED	1 TBSP BALSAMIC VINEGAR
1 TSP BLACK PEPPER	1 TBSP EXTRA VIRGIN OLIVE OIL
1/2 CUP ZUCCHINI, SLICED	2 SPRIGS THYME, TORN FROM THE STEM

---

1. Preheat the broiler to a medium-high heat.
2. Broil the salmon in parchment paper with the lemon juice and black pepper for 10 minutes.
3. Meanwhile, slice the zucchini and sauté with the greens for 4-5 minutes with the oil in a pan on a medium heat.
4. Build the salad by creating a bed of zucchini and topping with flaked salmon.
5. Drizzle with balsamic vinegar, olive oil and sprinkle with thyme.
6. Enjoy.

CUMIN & MANGO CHICKEN SALAD

SERVES 2   PREP TIME: 10 MINUTES   COOK TIME: 20 MINUTES

Spicy and refreshing all at the same time!

---

1 TBSP EXTRA VIRGIN OLIVE OIL

1 GARLIC CLOVE, MINCED

1 TSP OREGANO, FINELY CHOPPED

1 TSP CHILI FLAKES

1 TSP CUMIN

1 TSP TURMERIC

1 LIME, JUICED

2 FREE RANGE SKINLESS CHICKEN BREASTS

1 CUP MANGO, CUBED

1/2 ICEBERG/ROMAINE LETTUCE OR SIMILAR, SLICED

---

1. In a bowl mix oil, garlic, herbs and spices with the lime juice.
2. Add the chicken and marinate for as long as time permits.
3. When ready to serve, preheat the broiler to a medium-high heat.
4. Add the chicken to a lightly greased baking tray and broil for 15-20 minutes or until cooked through.
5. Combine the mango and lettuce in a serving bowl.
6. Once the chicken is cooked, serve immediately on top of the mango and lettuce.
7. Enjoy.

JAPANESE AVOCADO & SHRIMP SALAD

SERVES 2   PREP TIME: 15 MINUTES   COOK TIME: 10 MINUTES

Miso is a soy product with anti-inflammatory properties. Whilst it is high in sodium, it can be enjoyed as a symptom fighter every now and then.

1/2 TBSP EXTRA VIRGIN OLIVE OIL

1 GARLIC CLOVE, MINCED

2 CUPS OF RAW SHRIMP, WITH THE TAILS REMOVED

1/2 TSP CHILI POWDER

1/4 TSP CAYENNE

1 AVOCADO, SLICED

1/2 CUCUMBER, CHOPPED

2 CUPS SPINACH OR BABY KALE, WASHED AND CHOPPED

FOR THE MISO DRESSING:

1 THUMB SIZED PIECE OF FRESH GINGER, FINELY CHOPPED

2 TBSP EXTRA VIRGIN OLIVE OIL

3 TBSP LIME JUICE

2 TBSP AGAVE NECTAR/HONEY

1 TBSP WHITE MISO (AVAILABLE FROM MOST GROCERY STORES)

1/2 TSP MINCED GARLIC

1 TBSP CILANTRO, FRESHLY CHOPPED

1 TBSP PEANUTS, CRUSHED

1. Heat the oil in a skillet over a medium heat, adding in the garlic and shrimp, and then sprinkle with chili powder and cayenne.
2. Sauté for 8-10 minutes or until shrimp is cooked through.
3. Cut the avocado in half and scoop out the flesh.
4. Dice the cucumber, and chop the baby spinach/kale.
5. Arrange in a bowl with the cooked shrimp.
6. Put all of the ingredients for the dressing (up until minced garlic) into a food processor until smooth.
7. Pour over the salad and serve immediately, topping with cilantro and peanuts for an extra crunch.
8. Enjoy.

MACKEREL & BEETROOT SUPER SALAD

SERVES 2   PREP TIME: 5 MINUTES   COOK TIME: 20 MINUTES

Packed full of anti-inflammatory super foods, this is such a tasty lunch.

---

1 CUP SWEET POTATOES, PEELED

12 OZ SMOKED MACKEREL FILLETS, SKIN REMOVED

2 GREEN ONIONS, FINELY SLICED

1 CUP COOKED BEETS, SLICED INTO WEDGES

2 TBSP DILL, FINELY CHOPPED

2 TBSP OLIVE OIL

JUICE 1 LEMON, ZEST OF HALF

1 TSP CARAWAY SEEDS, CRUSHED USING PESTLE AND MORTAR

---

1. Place the potatoes in a pan of boiling water and simmer for 15 minutes on a medium-high heat or until fork-tender.
2. Cool and cut into thick slices.
3. Flake the mackerel into a bowl and add the cooled potatoes, green onions, beets and dill.
4. In a separate bowl, whisk together the olive oil, lemon juice, caraway seeds and black pepper.
5. Pour over the salad and toss well to coat.
6. Scatter over the lemon zest.
7. Pack into plastic containers and chill for later, or enjoy straight away.

MUSTARD & TARRAGON SWEET POTATO SALAD

SERVES 2   PREP TIME: 5 MINUTES   COOK TIME: 20 MINUTES

A BBQ favorite made the healthy way!

---

2 MEDIUM SIZED SWEET POTATOES, PEELED AND CUBED

1/2 CUP OF LOW-FAT GREEK YOGURT

2 TBSP OF DIJON MUSTARD

1 TBSP DRIED TARRAGON

1 BEEF TOMATO, FINELY CHOPPED (OPTIONAL)

1/2 YELLOW PEPPER, FINELY CHOPPED (OPTIONAL)

1/2 RED ONION, FINELY CHOPPED

PINCH OF BLACK PEPPER TO TASTE

---

1. Boil water in a large pot on a high heat.
2. Cook the potatoes in the pot for 20 minutes or until tender.
3. Set aside after draining to cool down.
4. Combine yogurt, Dijon mustard, tarragon, tomatoes, peppers, and red onion in a serving bowl.
5. Add the cooled potatoes and mix well.
6. Season with black pepper and enjoy!

EGG & MIXED BEAN SALAD

SERVES 4 / PREP TIME: 30 MINUTES / COOK TIME: NA

Classic American side dish.

1/2 CUP OF COOKED BLACK BEANS

1/2 CUP OF COOKED CANNELLINI BEANS

1/2 CUP OF COOKED KIDNEY BEANS

1 CELERY STICK, CHOPPED

2 GREEN ONIONS, CHOPPED

8 GREEN OLIVES, PITTED AND SLICED

1/2 TSP OF BLACK PEPPER

3 TSP EXTRA VIRGIN OLIVE OIL

1 TSP DRIED OREGANO

---

1. Rinse and drain the beans.
2. Combine the rest of the ingredients in a serving bowl.
3. Cover and refrigerate for at least 30 minutes.
4. Enjoy.

SIDES

HOMEMADE MOROCCAN HUMMUS

SERVES 4   PREP TIME: 10 MINUTES   COOK TIME: NA

Hummus is a great protein-rich snack straight from the Middle East which is now enjoyed across the world.

FOR THE HUMMUS:

1 CAN OF CHICKPEAS

2 CLOVES OF GARLIC, MINCED

1 TBSP TAHINI PASTE

4 TBSP EXTRA VIRGIN OLIVE OIL

1 TSP GROUND CUMIN

1 TSP TURMERIC

1 TSP HARISSA

1 TSP SALT

1 LEMON, JUICED

TO SERVE:

1/8 RED ONION, FINELY CHOPPED

1/2 BEEF TOMATO, FINELY CHOPPED (OPTIONAL)

1 TSP EXTRA VIRGIN OLIVE OIL

1. Take all of the ingredients for the hummus and add to a food processor until smooth (leave a little chunky for a rustic finish or add a little water to loosen the consistency if required).
2. Transfer to a serving dish and create a shallow well in the middle with your spoon.
3. Top with the mixed red onion and tomato and drizzle with the remaining oil to serve.
4. Sprinkle with a little black pepper to taste and serve as a dip for your favorite veggies or even as a side with quinoa or favorite fish or meat dish.

TARRAGON SWEDE AND CARROT MASH

SERVES 4   PREP TIME: 5 MINUTES   COOK TIME: 15 MINUTES

Try this home comfort – it's exciting mash!

---

4 CARROTS, CHOPPED

1/2 SWEDE, CHOPPED

3 GARLIC CLOVES, CHOPPED

1/4 CUP TARRAGON, FINELY CHOPPED

1 TBSP EXTRA VIRGIN OLIVE OIL

A PINCH OF BLACK PEPPER

1 TBSP LOW FAT GREEK YOGURT

---

1. Add the carrots, swede and garlic to a large pan of water, bring to the boil, and cook for 15 minutes. Drain.
2. Add the tarragon and olive oil and season with pepper.
3. Mash with a potato masher.
4. Stir in a dollop of low fat Greek yogurt if desired.
5. Serve and enjoy!

SUPER HEALTHY SWEET POTATO FRIES

SERVES 2   PREP TIME: 5 MINUTES   COOK TIME: 30 MINUTES

A healthy version of a favorite snack – enjoy without the guilt!

---

2 LARGE SWEET POTATOES, CUT INTO THIN STRIPS

1 TBSP OF EXTRA VIRGIN OLIVE OIL

1 TSP OF CUMIN

1/2 TSP OF BLACK PEPPER

1/2 TSP OF PAPRIKA

1 DASH OF CAYENNE PEPPER

---

1. Preheat oven to 375°F/190 °C/Gas Mark 5.
2. Add the sweet potato strips into a large bowl.
3. Drizzle with olive oil.
4. Sprinkle the rest of the ingredients over the top.
5. Toss together gently to evenly coat the potatoes.
6. Get a baking sheet and arrange the coated potatoes into a thin layer.
7. Bake for around 30 minutes or until cooked through.
8. Serve.

CAYENNE-SPICED BEANS & SWEET POTATO

SERVES 4   PREP TIME: 5 MINUTES   COOK TIME: 30 MINUTES

This is a healthy and tasty rice dish.

---

1 TBSP EXTRA VIRGIN OLIVE OIL

2 CLOVES OF GARLIC, MINCED

1/2 ONION, DICED

2 MEDIUM CARROTS, SLICED

2 SWEET POTATOES, PEELED & CHOPPED

1 CAN BLACK BEANS

1 CAN CANNELLINI BEANS

1 CAN CHOPPED TOMATOES

1 CUP VEGETABLE BROTH
1 TBSP CHILI POWDER

1/2 TSP GARLIC POWDER

1 TSP CUMIN

1/2 TSP CAYENNE

1/2 TSP SALT

1/2 TSP BLACK PEPPER

---

1. Heat olive oil in a pan over a medium heat.
2. Sauté garlic and onions for 1-2 minutes.
3. Add carrots and sweet potatoes for about 6 minutes or until the onions are soft.
4. Lower heat setting to medium-low, then add the rest of the ingredients.
5. Cover partially and simmer for around 25 minutes, occasionally stirring to prevent sticking.
6. Serve hot and enjoy.

MEXICAN SPICE INFUSED QUINOA

SERVES 1   PREP TIME: 5 MINUTES   COOK TIME:30 MINUTES

A spicy Mexican side dish.

1 TSP OLIVE OIL	1 CAN DICED TOMATOES
1 CUP RINSED QUINOA	1 TBSP PAPRIKA
1 WHITE ONION, DICED	2 CUPS LOW-SALT CHICKEN BROTH
2 CLOVES GARLIC, MINCED	1 TBSP FRESH CILANTRO, CHOPPED
1 JALAPEÑO, CHOPPED	1 LIME, JUICED
1 CHILI PEPPER, DICED	1/2 CUP CILANTRO

1. Heat the oil in a skillet and cook the quinoa and onion in the oil for 5 minutes or until the onion becomes translucent.
2. Add the garlic, jalapeño and pepper and cook for 4-5 minutes until the garlic is fragrant.
3. Mix the undrained can of tomatoes with the paprika, and the chicken broth into the garlic and pepper.
4. Turn up heat to bring to the boil, then turn heat down to medium and allow to simmer for about 15-20 minutes, until the liquid reduces.
5. Stir in the cilantro and lime juice and serve.

TASTY TURNIP CHIPS

SERVES 4   PREP TIME: 5 MINUTES   COOK TIME: 50 MINUTES

Lightly spiced turnip side.

---

1 TBSP EXTRA VIRGIN OLIVE OIL

1 RUTABAGA, PEELED AND FINELY SLICED

1 TURNIP, PEELED AND FINELY SLICED

1 ONION, CHOPPED

1 CLOVE GARLIC, MINCED

1 TSP BLACK PEPPER

1 TSP OREGANO

1 TSP PAPRIKA

---

1. Heat oven to 375°f/190°c/Gas Mark 5.
2. Grease a baking tray with a little olive oil
3. Add turnip and rutabaga in a thin layer.
4. Dust over herbs and spices.
5. Drizzle over the rest of the olive oil.
6. Bake for 40-50 minutes (turning half way through to ensure even crispiness!)
7. Serve with your choice of low fat Greek yogurt, tomato sauce or mustard.
8. Enjoy.

GINGER PURPLE SPROUTING BROCCOLI

SERVES 2   PREP TIME: 2 MINUTES   COOK TIME: 10 MINUTES

Packing a punch.

**2 CUPS OF TENDER STEM BROCCOLI OR
PURPLE SPROUTING BROCCOLI**

1 TBSP EXTRA VIRGIN OLIVE OIL

**1 THUMB SIZED PIECE OF GINGER,
PEELED AND MINCED**

---

1. Boil water in a medium sized pan and steam the broccoli for about 5 minutes or until tender and crisp.
2. Drain and transfer to ice cold water to preserve the nutrients.
3. In a skillet, heat the oil for 30 seconds and then stir-fry the ginger for 15 seconds, mix in the broccoli, and sauté for 3 minutes until hot throughout.
4. Serve as a delicious snack or on the side of your favorite meal and enjoy.

SPINACH & KALE BREADED BALLS

SERVES 4   PREP TIME: 5 MINUTES   COOK TIME: 30 MINUTES

These can be prepared in advance and then heated to serve and are packed with vitamins and iron.

---

3 TBSP EXTRA VIRGIN OLIVE OIL

2 FREE RANGE EGGS, BEATEN

2 CUPS FROZEN OR FRESH SPINACH, THAWED AND CHOPPED

1 CUP OF FROZEN OR FRESH KALE, THAWED AND DRAINED

1/2 CUP ONION, FINELY CHOPPED

1 GARLIC CLOVE, FINELY CHOPPED

1/2 TSP GROUND THYME

1/2 TSP RUBBED DRIED OREGANO

1/2 TSP DRIED ROSEMARY

1 CUP DRY 100% WHOLEGRAIN BREAD CRUMBS (GF)

1/2 TSP DRIED OREGANO

1 TSP GROUND BLACK PEPPER

---

1. Preheat oven to 350°f/170°c/Gas Mark 4.
2. Line a baking sheet with parchment paper.
3. In a bowl, mix the olive oil and eggs, adding in the spinach, kale, onion and garlic and tossing to coat.
4. Add the rest of the ingredients, mixing to blend.
5. Use the palms of your hands to roll into 1 inch balls and arrange them onto the baking sheet.
6. Bake for 15 minutes, and then flip the balls over.
7. Continue to bake for another 15 minutes or until they're golden brown.
8. Serve with low fat Greek yogurt or on their own.
9. Enjoy.

CARROT & TART CHERRY KETCHUP

SERVES 2   PREP TIME: 5 MINUTES   COOK TIME: 20 MINUTES

Sweet and savory - give it a go!

---

5 CARROTS, PEELED AND SLICED

1/2 CUP DRIED TART CHERRIES

---

1. Boil a pan of water on a high heat.
2. Boil carrots for 10 minutes and then remove and set aside in a separate bowl.
3. Add the cherries to the water and cook for a further 10 minutes before draining.
4. Blend carrots and cherries in a blender until puréed.
5. Serve as a dip or drizzled over a summer salad and enjoy.

MUSTARD CAULIFLOWER SLICES

SERVES 2   PREP TIME: 5 MINUTES   COOK TIME: 0 MINUTES

Raw cauliflower has double the amount of Vitamin B6 and potassium than cooked cauliflower and tastes amazing.

---

2 CUPS CAULIFLOWER FLORETS, FINELY SLICED

FOR THE DRESSING:

1 TSP EXTRA VIRGIN OLIVE OIL

1 LEMON, JUICED

1 LARGE GARLIC CLOVE, MINCED

1 TSP WHOLEGRAIN MUSTARD

---

1. Make your dressing by whisking ingredients together.
1. Get a large salad bowl and combine all of the ingredients.
2. Serve immediately so that the cauliflower remains crunchy!
3. Enjoy.

CASHEW NUTS & BROCCOLI SNACK

SERVES 4   PREP TIME: 5 MINUTES   COOK TIME: 25 MINUTES

This is a simple and flavorsome salad.

1/2 CUP CASHEWS

4 CUPS BROCCOLI, FLORETS

1/2 CUP WATER

2 TBSP YELLOW CURRY POWDER

PINCH OF PEPPER

2 TBSP SUNFLOWER SEEDS

---

1. Preheat oven to the highest heat.
2. Layer the cashew nuts onto a dry baking tray and add to the oven for 5-10 minutes or until nuts start to brown. Turn whilst cooking to ensure even browning.
3. Remove to cool.
4. Meanwhile boil a pan of water on a medium heat and add the broccoli.
5. Cook on a simmer for 5-10 minutes or until cooked through.
6. Drain and place to one side.
7. Whisk together the rest of the ingredients.
8. Crush the cashew nuts on a wooden chopping board or similar, using a sharp knife.
9. When ready to serve, dress the broccoli with the sesame dressing, and top with roasted cashew nuts.
10. Enjoy.

TUNA & BLACK OLIVE TAPENADE

SERVES 2   PREP TIME: 5 MINUTES   COOK TIME: 0 MINUTES

This quick and easy tapanade can be served on a bed of salad or as a dip.

---

1 GARLIC CLOVE

1/2 CUP OF SMALL BLACK OLIVES, DRAINED

1/2 CUP CAPERS, RINSED AND DRAINED

4 ANCHOVIES

1 TBSP DIJON MUSTARD

4 TBSP OF EXTRA VIRGIN OLIVE OIL

1 CAN OF TUNA IN SPRING WATER, DRAINED

1 CUP WATERCRESS

---

1. Combine all ingredients down to the mustard with 2 tbsp olive oil to a food processor for 30 seconds or until a paste is formed.
2. Transfer to a separate bowl and add 2 tbsp olive oil - do not stir.
3. Add the tuna to the tapanade and mix well.
4. Serve on a bed of watercress and enjoy.

BRILLIANT BEET KETCHUP

SERVES 2   PREP TIME: 5 MINUTES   COOK TIME: 45 MINUTES

Vibrant and enticing.

---

2 WHOLE BEETS

1 JUICED LEMON

4 TBSP SUNFLOWER SEEDS, SOAKED OVERNIGHT

1 TSP MUSTARD POWDER

A PINCH OF BLACK PEPPER TO TASTE

---

1. Preheat oven 350°F/180 °C/Gas Mark 4.
2. Bake the beetroot for 30-40 minutes or until tender, and then peel and chop into cubes.
3. Add the rest of the ingredients and the beetroot into a blender and puree until smooth.
4. You can use prepared beetroot as a shortcut as long as it contains no added sugar or salt (check the package).

ZANY ZUCCHINI KETCHUP

SERVES 4   PREP TIME: 15 MINUTES   COOK TIME: NA

A yummy alternative to tomato ketchup!

---

2 ZUCCHINIS, PEELED AND SLICED

1/2 CUP FRESH PARSLEY

2 TBSP LEMON JUICE

1 TBSP EXTRA VIRGIN OLIVE OIL

1 GARLIC CLOVE, MINCED

A PINCH OF BLACK PEPPER

2 TBSP CHOPPED WALNUTS

---

1. Allow zucchini to dry out a little by slicing and placing on kitchen towel to soak up the moisture for 10 minutes or longer if possible.
2. Process the zucchini with the rest of the ingredients (apart from the nuts) until smooth.
3. Fold the nuts into the mixture and then refrigerate for at least 10 minutes before serving with your favorite crudités or sweet potato fries.
4. Enjoy.

LEMONY TARO DIP

SERVES 4   PREP TIME: 5 MINUTES   COOK TIME: NA

This is a great dip for a snack or dinner.

GARLIC CLOVE, PEELED

3 CUPS OF TARO (RETAIN THE WATER IT WAS COOKED IN)

2 TBSP LEMON JUICE

2 TBSP EXTRA VIRGIN OLIVE OIL

1/2 CUP FRESH PARSLEY

1/2 CUP TOASTED PINE NUTS

A PINCH OF BLACK PEPPER

---

1. In a blender, process the garlic and then add in the taro, lemon juice, olive oil and the water and blend for about 10 seconds.
2. Transfer to a serving dish and garnish with the parsley, pine nuts and pepper.
3. Enjoy as a dip for crudités or wholemeal pita bread.

FARRO & TOMATO PILAF

SERVES 4   PREP TIME: 5 MINUTES   COOK TIME: 20 MINUTES

An Indian inspired side dish.

---

1 CUP PEARLED FARRO, RINSED

2 CUPS WATER

1 CUP TOMATOES, CHOPPED

1 PACKAGE FRESH MUSHROOMS, SLICED

1 TBSP CILANTRO

1 TSP CUMIN

1 TSP CHILI POWDER

1 TSP TURMERIC

1/2 YELLOW SQUASH, CUBED

---

1. Add the faro and water to a saucepan and boil on a high heat until boiling.
2. Reduce the heat, cover and simmer for 20 minutes or until the farro is tender and the liquid is absorbed.
3. Meanwhile, in a separate pan on a medium heat, cook the tomatoes and mushrooms with the cilantro and spices until the mushrooms are soft (5 minutes).
4. Add the squash and sauté for 10 minutes or until all of the vegetables are tender.
5. Drain and stir the farro into the squash mix until heated through.
6. Serve alone as lunch or on the side of your favorite dish.
7. Enjoy.

RUSTIC APRICOT & WALNUT RICE

SERVES 2   PREP TIME: 5 MINUTES   COOK TIME: 25 MINUTES

A sweet and savory side.

1/2 CUP WALNUTS

2 CUPS HOMEMADE CHICKEN BROTH

1 CUP UNCOOKED BROWN RICE

1 TBSP EXTRA VIRGIN OLIVE OIL

1 ONION, CHOPPED

1/2 CUP DRIED APRICOTS

1 ORANGE, ZEST AND JUICE

---

1. Preheat oven to 375°F/190 °C/Gas Mark 5.
2. Layer walnuts on a baking tray and roast for 10 minutes.
3. Meanwhile, put the broth and brown rice into a saucepan and boil on a high heat.
4. Reduce the heat and simmer for 25 minutes until rice is cooked and the broth is absorbed.
5. Meanwhile, heat the oil in a skillet on a medium heat and sauté the onion until soft.
6. Add the apricots and cook for another 10 minutes.
7. Stir in the walnuts and the orange zest and juice, and then fold the mixture into the rice, adding pepper to taste.
8. Enjoy hot or cold.

ROASTED PAPRIKA PUMPKIN SEEDS

SERVES 4   PREP TIME: 5 MINUTES   COOK TIME: 15 MINUTES

Energy boosting bites – great as a topping for cereals or soups, or as a quick pick me up throughout the day!

1 CUP PUMPKIN SEEDS

1 TBSP EXTRA VIRGIN OLIVE OIL

1 TSP PAPRIKA

1 TSP CHILI POWDER

1 TSP DRIED OREGANO

1. Preheat oven to 375°F/190 °C/Gas Mark 5.
2. Layer the seeds on a baking tray.
3. Combine the oil, paprika, chili powder and oregano together and then pour over the pumpkin seeds.
4. Toss to coat.
5. Bake for 15 minutes and serve alone or top your favorite salad or vegetables with them!
6. Enjoy.

FAST & FRESH GRANOLA TRAIL MIX

SERVES 2   PREP TIME: 5 MINUTES   COOK TIME: 20 MINUTES

This is a tasty granola filled with protein and so much healthier than the shop bought version.

1 CUP TOASTED ALMONDS	1 CUP WHOLEGRAIN OATS (GF)
1/2 CUP CHERRIES	1 TBSP RAW HONEY

1. Preheat oven to 350°F/170 °C/Gas Mark 4.
2. Spread the almonds across a baking sheet.
3. Bake for five minutes and then add cherries and oats and toss.
4. Drizzle honey on top and toss again to coat before baking in oven for 10-15 minutes.
5. Remove to cool.
6. Serve alone or with your choice of milk as a cereal and enjoy.

BAKED APPLE & WALNUT CHIPS

SERVES 4   PREP TIME: 5 MINUTES   COOK TIME: 30 MINUTES

These chips will satisfy your sweet cravings without flaring up symptoms!

---

4 APPLES, PEELED AND THINLY SLICED

1 TBSP CINNAMON

1/4 CUP OF WALNUT PIECES FOR TOPPING

---

1. Preheat oven to 190°C/375°F/Gas Mark 5.
2. Layer the apple slices in a thin layer on a baking tray.
3. Dust with the cinnamon and top with walnut pieces.
4. Bake for 20-30 minutes or until crispy.
5. Enjoy.

DESSERTS

WALNUT & DARK CHOCOLATE CHIP COOKIES

SERVES 5   PREP TIME: 10 MINUTES   COOK TIME: 10 MINUTES

These wholegrain cookies are just as delicious as their sugary companions! .

---

1 CUP WALNUTS/PECANS

1 CUP GROUND FLAX MEAL

2 CUPS WHOLEGRAIN ROLLED OATS

1 TSP CINNAMON

1/2 CUP WHOLE WHEAT FLOUR (GF)

1 TSP BAKING SODA

1/4 CUP STEVIA

1 FREE RANGE EGG

1/4 CUP CANOLA OIL

1 TSP VANILLA EXTRACT

1 CUP DARK CHOCOLATE CHIPS

1/2 CUP DRIED TART CHERRIES

1/2 CUP WHOLE ALMOND BUTTER

---

1. Preheat the oven to 190°C/375°F/Gas Mark 5.
2. Line a baking dish with parchment paper.
3. Grind the walnuts in a blender to make flour.
4. Add all of the other ingredients (except for the almond butter, cherries and chocolate chips) and process.
5. Add mixture to a bowl and then fold in the chocolate chips and cherries.
6. Mix the flour mixture into the almond butter until a sticky dough is formed.
7. Use a tablespoon to spoon mini cookie shapes onto your baking tray and bake for 9 minutes before placing them on a wire rack to cool.
8. Enjoy.

STRAWBERRY & BANANA PUDDING

SERVES 2   PREP TIME: 30 MINUTES   COOK TIME: 5 MINUTES

Summery and scrumptious!

---

4 SQUARES DARK CHOCOLATE

2 TBSP OF WATER

1/4 CUP OF FREE RANGE EGG WHITES

1 CUP OF STRAWBERRIES, SLICED

1 SMALL BANANA, SLICED

1/2 CUP BLUEBERRIES

---

1. Break the dark chocolate into squares and add to a glass heat-proof bowl.
2. Place this over a pan of boiling water and stir the chocolate until melted.
3. Remove the bowl from the heat.
4. Add the water and egg whites to the melted chocolate and mix well to reach a thick consistency.
5. Spoon the batter out into 2 ramekins.
6. Put in the freezer for half an hour.
7. Garnish with the fresh fruit to serve and enjoy.

VANILLA, NUTMEG & BLUEBERRY MUFFINS

SERVES 4   PREP TIME: 10 MINUTES   COOK TIME: 20 MINUTES

Scrumptious muffins to be enjoyed as a delicious dessert or breakfast!

---

3 FREE RANGE EGG WHITES

1/10 CUP CHICKPEA FLOUR

1 TBSP COCONUT FLOUR

1 TSP OF BAKING POWDER

1 TBSP NUTMEG, GRATED

1 TSP VANILLA EXTRACT

1 TSP STEVIA

1/2 CUP FRESH BLUEBERRIES

---

1. Preheat the oven to 325°F/170 °C/Gas Mark 3.
2. Lightly oil a 4 case muffin tin.
3. Mix all of the ingredients in a large mixing bowl.
4. Divide the batter into 4 and spoon into a muffin cases.
5. Bake in the oven for 15-20 minutes or until cooked through.
6. Your knife should pull out clean from the middle of the muffins once done.
7. Allow to cool on a wired rack before serving.
8. Enjoy.

HOMEMADE HOT CROSS BUNS

SERVES 6   PREP TIME: 10 MINUTES   COOK TIME: 20 MINUTES

Anti-inflammatory friendly treats.

---

3 CUPS ALMONDS

1 TBSP RAW HONEY

1 TSP CINNAMON

1 TSP CLOVES

1 TSP NUTMEG

ZEST AND JUICE OF 1 ORANGE AND 1 LEMON

1 CUP RAISINS

---

1. Lightly oil a 6 case muffin tray.
2. Blend the almonds into a powder in a food processor until a fine powder is formed.
3. Add the honey, spices, lemon juice and orange juice and process until you have a dough.
4. You can then blend in the raisins and the fruit zest for about 30 seconds.
5. Divide mixture into the muffin cases and then cross the top of each bun with a sharp knife.
6. Add to the oven for 15-20 minutes or until risen and cooked through.
7. These should be served immediately and enjoyed with your favorite fresh fruit.

SPICED ORANGES

SERVES 2   PREP TIME: 20 MINUTES   COOK TIME: 15 MINUTES

These oranges are delicious all year round.

1/2 CUP WATER	1 SMALL CINNAMON STICK
1 TBSP RAW HONEY	1 CLOVE
1 LEMON	1 SPRIG OF FRESH MINT
	2 ORANGES, PEELED AND SECTIONED

---

1. Add all of the ingredients (except the oranges) to a saucepan.
2. Cook over a medium heat until thickened (10-15 minutes).
3. Add the oranges, and then simmer for 1 minute.
4. Transfer all ingredients to a bowl or container and place in the fridge, marinating for at least 2 hours or preferably overnight.
5. Drain orange slices and garnish with a little more fresh mint to serve.
6. Best served with low fat Greek yogurt for summer or warmed through in the winter.

FRUIT COCKTAIL & ROSE WATER YOGURT

SERVES 4　PREP TIME: 10 MINUTES　COOK TIME: NA
A timeless treat!

---

2 CUPS FRESH STRAWBERRIES, HALVED

2 PLUMS, PITTED AND CUBED

2 KIWIS, PEELED AND CUBED

1 PEACH, PEELED AND CUBED

1 CUP HONEYDEW MELON, PEELED AND CUBED

1 CUP OF TART CHERRIES, PITTED AND HALVED

1 CUP GRAPES, HALVED

1 CUP FRESH PINEAPPLE, CUBED

1 TBSP ROSE WATER (AVAILABLE IN MOST EXOTIC AISLES IN GROCERY STORES, ALTERNATIVELY USE 1-2 DROPS OF ROSE OIL)

2 CUPS LOW-FAT GREEK YOGURT (OPTIONAL)

---

1. Add all of the fruit to a mixing bowl and stir.
2. In a separate bowl, add rose water to yogurt and stir.
3. Divide fruit into 4 servings and top with rose water yogurt.
4. Enjoy!

DELICIOUS DATE & APPLE COMPOTE

SERVES 2   PREP TIME: 1 HOUR   COOK TIME: 10 MINUTES

Rich and satisfying.

---

2 CUPS OF DATES, FINELY CHOPPED

2 CUPS DRIED APRICOTS, FINELY CHOPPED

2 CUPS BLACK FIGS, FINELY CHOPPED

2 CUPS DRIED PEACHES, FINELY CHOPPED

4 CUPS APPLES,

1 LEMON

---

1. Add fruit to a large pan and cover with water.
2. Soak the fruit for an hour and then bring to a boil on a high heat.
3. Turn down the heat and simmer for 5 minutes.
4. Add the juice of 1 lemon and stir.
5. Remove from the heat and allow to cool.
6. Blend in a food processor if needed to smooth any lumps.
7. Serve warm on the side of any dessert.
8. Enjoy.

BAKED FRUIT & NUT PUDDING

SERVES 2   PREP TIME: 5 MINUTES   COOK TIME: 1 HOUR

Scrumptious.

---

3 CUPS WATER

15 APRICOTS

10 PRUNES

2 CINNAMON STICKS

6 FREE RANGE EGGS

2 TBSP PURE VANILLA EXTRACT

1 CUP RAW PECANS/WALNUTS

---

1. Preheat oven to 180°C/350°F/Gas Mark 4.
2. In a large saucepan, boil the water on a high heat and then add the apricots, prunes and cinnamon sticks before turning down the heat and simmering for 30 minutes.
3. Allow to cool.
4. Remove the cinnamon sticks, drain and blend fruit in a food processor, adding in the eggs and vanilla until smooth.
5. Add mixture to an glass oven dish and layer the top with the nuts.
6. Oven bake for 30 minutes.
7. Cool and serve.

GRILLED BANANA & NUT BUTTER

SERVES 2   PREP TIME: 5 MINUTES   COOK TIME: 30 MINUTES

Loaded with goodness for a mid afternoon snack!

---

2 BANANAS

2 TBSP ALMOND BUTTER (CHECK LABEL TO ENSURE THERE ARE NO EXTRA IN-GREDIENTS)

---

1. Split bananas lengthwise with a knife down the center to form a banana split.
2. Spread almond butter along the middle and broil for 3-4 minutes under broiler on a medium heat until browned.
3. Serve immediately – this is just as tasty cold if you're in a rush!
4. Enjoy.

APRICOT & COCONUT BITES

SERVES 2   PREP TIME: 30 MINUTES   COOK TIME: NA

Tropical dessert.

SUN-DRIED APRICOTS, FINELY CHOPPED

RAW WALNUTS OR PECANS, FINELY CHOPPED

1/2 CUP DESICCATED COCONUT

1 TBSP HONEY

---

1. Mix all the ingredients together to form a sticky dough.
2. Shape it into bite size balls with the palms of your hands.
3. Cover and refrigerate for at least 2 hours to set.
4. Enjoy.

COCONUT, BANANA & RASPBERRY HOT MILK

SERVES 2   PREP TIME: 5 MINUTES   COOK TIME: 5 MINUTES

A hot drink full of fruity flavor.

---

1 CAN LOW FAT COCONUT MILK

1 BANANA, SLICED

1/2CUP FRESH RASPBERRIES

---

1. Add all of the ingredients to a blender or smoothie maker until smooth.
1. Add to a pan over a medium-low heat.
2. Simmer until hot through.
3. Serve warm or allow to cool and add ice cubes to serve as a chilled milkshake.
4. Enjoy.

SPICED PUMPKIN PANCAKES

SERVES 2   PREP TIME: 5 MINUTES   COOK TIME: 10 MINUTES

Savory pancakes for those of us who don't have a sweet tooth!

FLESH FROM 1/4 DE-SEEDED PUMPKIN

4 EGGS (FREE RANGE)

3 EGG WHITES (FREE RANGE)

SPRINKLE OF BLACK PEPPER

2 TBSP COCONUT OIL

1/2 TSP GLUTEN-FREE BAKING SODA

1 HANDFUL PECAN NUTS

1 TBSP GOOD QUALITY MAPLE SYRUP

---

1. In a blender or food processor, blend the pumpkin flesh together with 2 tbsp of water to form a smooth pulp.
2. Now add the eggs and egg whites, freshly ground pepper, 1 tbsp of coconut oil, and baking soda to the pumpkin mix, blend until smooth.
3. Heat a large pan on a medium heat with the other tbsp of coconut oil.
4. Into the pan, pour individual rounded pancakes (go easy at first and pour your mixture into little circles, keep pouring whilst tilting the pan until you have a pancake to your desired shape).
5. Lift the mixture with a spatula and then flip.
6. Cook for 3 minutes on either side.
7. Plate and serve with pecan nuts and maple syrup.

PEANUT CEREAL BARS

SERVES 4-6   PREP TIME: 5 MINUTES   COOK TIME: 30 MINUTES

Save your money with these homemade cereal bars - they're delicious!

1/2 CUP COCONUT MILK

1 CUP ALMOND BUTTER

2 CUPS OF WHOLEGRAIN OATS (GF)

---

1. Whisk the coconut milk in a mixing bowl until smooth.
2. Add the almond butter and mix thoroughly.
3. Pour the oats into the bowl and mix through.
4. Scoop out the mixture onto a baking tray and flatten until the surface is smooth.
5. Place the tray in the fridge and leave for around 8 hours.
6. Cut into bars 4-5 bars and serve.

FRUIT & NUT SLICES

SERVES 2   PREP TIME: 5 MINUTES   COOK TIME: 30 MINUTES

Sweet and savory treat.

---

1 TBSP DRIED DATES, DICED

1 TBSP DRIED CRANBERRIES

1 TBSP COCONUT FLAKES

1 TBSP WALNUTS/PECANS, GROUND

---

1. Mix all of the ingredients in a mixing bowl.
2. Use your hands to shape the mixture into a ball.
3. Lay out tin foil and then flatten and roll the mixture with the palms of your hands to form a cylinder shape.
4. Roll and wrap in the tinfoil and then leave it in the fridge for 30 minutes until it hardens before slicing into disk shape slices and serving with some fresh fruit or yogurt.
5. Enjoy.

PEANUT CHOCOLATE PANCAKES

SERVES 2   PREP TIME: 5 MINUTES   COOK TIME: 10 MINUTES

Much better than your average candy bar.

---

2 TBSP OF SMOOTH PEANUT BUTTER

2 SQUARES OF DARK CHOCOLATE, GRATED

2 FREE RANGE EGG WHITES

2 TBSP OF RAW COCONUT FLOUR

1 TBSP COCONUT OIL

---

1. Get a bowl and combine all the ingredients (except the coconut oil).
2. Mix well to form a thick batter.
3. Heat a skillet over a medium heat and add the coconut oil.
4. Pour half the mixture onto the center of the pan, to form a pancake and cook through for 3-4 minutes on each side.
5. Serve with your choice of berry or Greek yogurt and enjoy.

LAVENDER & STRAWBERRY COMPOTE

SERVES 4   PREP TIME: 5 MINUTES   COOK TIME: 30 MINUTES

So sweet and delicious.

JUICE AND ZEST OF 1 LEMON

2 TBSP RAW HONEY

1 TBSP LAVENDER EXTRACT

2 CUPS OF STRAWBERRIES, HALVED

1. Put all of the ingredients together into a saucepan (except for strawberries) and then simmer on a very low heat until the honey has been dissolved (15-20 minutes).
2. When the sauce starts to thicken, add the strawberries and simmer for 5-10 minutes.
3. Serve warm right away or allow to cool and drizzle over yogurt later on.
4. Enjoy.

PECAN & DATE SNACK BARS

SERVES 4   PREP TIME: 20 MINUTES   COOK TIME: 40 MINUTES

These are great protein bars for on the go healthy snacking!

---

4 CUPS OF DATES, PITTED & CHOPPED

3 CUPS PECANS

---

1. Preheat the oven to 180°C/350°F/Gas Mark 4.
2. Put the dates in a bowl and cover with warm water.
3. Leave for at least 20 minutes and then blitz the pecans in a food processor until they form a 'breadcrumb' texture.
4. Now, drain the water from the dates and add to the processor until the nuts and fruit create a dough that easily needs together with your hands.
5. Line a baking sheet with parchment paper and then spread the dough onto the pan into a layer 2 inches thick.
6. Bake for 35-40 minutes or until cooked through and crispy on the top.
7. Remove to cool and slice into bars to serve.
8. Enjoy.

SUNSHINE CEREAL BITES

SERVES 2   PREP TIME: 20 MINUTES   COOK TIME: 30 MINUTES

You can't stay dreary and sad with these delectable fruit bites!

---

1 CUP UNSWEETENED PINEAPPLE, DRIED   1 TBSP HONEY

1/2 CUP WARM WATER

1 CUP CASHEWS

1/2 CUP COCONUT FLAKES

1/2 TSP LEMON ZEST

---

1. Preheat oven to 190°C/375°F/Gas Mark 5.
2. Soak the pineapple slices in 2 cups of warm water for 20 minutes until softened.
3. Combine with the rest of the ingredients and mix.
4. Spread onto a lined baking tray and bake for 20-30 minutes or until crispy.
5. Allow to cool.
6. Slice up and enjoy.

CONVERSION TABLES

Volume

Imperial	Metric
1 tbsp	15ml
2 fl oz	55 ml
3 fl oz	75 ml
5 fl oz (¼ pint)	150 ml
10 fl oz (½ pint)	275 ml
1 pint	570 ml
1 ¼ pints	725 ml
1 ¾ pints	1 litre
2 pints	1.2 litres
2½ pints	1.5 litres
4 pints	2.25 litres

Oven temperatures

Gas Mark	Fahrenheit	Celsius
1/4	225	110
1/2	250	130
1	275	140
2	300	150
3	325	170
4	350	180
5	375	190
6	400	200
7	425	220
8	450	230
9	475	240

Weight

Imperial	Metric
½ oz	10 g
¾ oz	20 g
1 oz	25 g
1½ oz	40 g
2 oz	50 g
2½ oz	60 g
3 oz	75 g
4 oz	110 g
4½ oz	125 g
5 oz	150 g
6 oz	175 g
7 oz	200 g
8 oz	225 g
9 oz	250 g
10 oz	275 g

BIBLIOGRAPHY

Beck, S. (2013) Acute and Chronic Information. [online] Hopkins Medicine. Available at: http://www.hopkinsmedicine.org/mcp/education/300.713%20lectures/300.713%202013/beck_08.26.2013.pdf Accessed 03/04/2016

Women's Health, (2012). Auto-immune Diseases Fact Sheet. Available at: http://www.womenshealth.gov/publications/our-publications/fact-sheet/autoimmune-diseases.html#a Accessed 04/03/2016

MACKAY, I AND ROSEN, F. (2001) Autoimmune Diseases. The New England Journal of Medicine [online] Vol. 345, No. 5, · www.nejm.org. [Accessed 07/02/2016]

US National Library of Medicine (2014) Multiple Sclerosis. Available at: https://www.nlm.nih.gov/medlineplus/ency/article/000737.htm [Accessed 04/03/2016]

Cosentino, F and Assenza, E. (December 2004), Diabetes and Inflammation. Herz. Volume 29, Issue 8, pp 749-759 [Accessed 07/02/2016]

Baecklund, E and Anastasia, L. (February 2006), Arthritis & Rheumatism. Volume 54, Issue 3, pages 692–701, [Accessed 07/02/2016] Xu, Haiyan et al. "Chronic Inflammation In Fat Plays A Crucial Role In The Development Of Obesity-Related Insulin Resistance". Journal of Clinical Investigation 112.12 (2003): 1821-1830. Web. [Accessed 07/02/2016]

Shacter, E and Weitzman, SA (2002) Chronic inflammation and cancer. Oncology (Williston Park, N.Y.) Volume 16, Issue 2. pp. 217-26, 229 [Accessed 07/02/2016]

Galland, L. "Diet And Inflammation". Nutrition in Clinical Practice 25.6 (2010): 634-640. Web. [Accessed 02/01/2016] Bernhard Watz (2013) Anti-inflammatory Effects of Plant-based Foods and of their Constituents, International Journal for Vitamin and Nutrition Research, Volume 78, pp. 293-298. [Accessed 01/20/2016]

Adam, O et al. (January 2003), Anti-inflammatory effects of a low arachidonic acid diet and fish oil in patients with rheumatoid arthritis, Rheumatology International, Volume 23, Issue 1, pp 27-36 [Accessed 09/03/2016]

www.nutrition.org [Accessed 02/03/2016]

Grzanna, L et al (2005). Ginger—An Herbal Medicinal Product with Broad Anti-Inflammatory Actions, Journal of Medicinal Food. Volume 8, Issue 2: pp. 125-132. [Accessed 01/01/2016] Arthritis.org. 8 Food Ingredients That Can Cause Inflammation. Available at: http://www.arthritis.org/living-with-arthritis/arthritis-diet/foods-to-avoid-limit/food-ingredients-and-inflammation-12.php [Accessed on 03/29/2016]

NIH (2014) Handout on Health: Rheumatoid Arthritis. Available at: http://www.niams.nih.gov/Health_Info/Rheumatic_Disease/ [Accessed on 04/03/2016]

INDEX

Made in the USA
Middletown, DE
16 April 2019